THE NURSE'S QUEST FOR
A PROFESSIONAL IDENTITY

THE NURSE'S QUEST FOR
A PROFESSIONAL IDENTITY

Helen A. Cohen, Ph.D.
Director of Psychological Services,
Cook County School of Nursing, Chicago, Illinois

⚛ **Addison-Wesley Publishing Company**
Medical/Nursing Division • Menlo Park, California
Reading, Massachusetts • London • Amsterdam
Don Mills, Ontario • Sydney

Sponsoring Editor: Pat Franklin
Production Coordinator: Madeleine Dreyfack
Production Editor: Nancy Sjoberg
Cover Designer: Michael Rogondino
Book Designer: Deborah Gale

Library of Congress Cataloging in Publication Data

Cohen, Helen A   1932-

    The nurse's quest for a professional identity.

    Bibliography: p. 188
    Includes index.
    1. Nursing — Study and teaching — Social
aspects — United States. 2. Nursing students —
United States. 3. Professional socialization.
I. Title [DNLM: 1. Socialization. 2. Nurses.
3. Education, Nursing. WY16 C678s]
RT79.C63   610.73'07'1   80-22336
ISBN 0-201-00956-0
    0-201-01157-3 (pbk.)

ABCDEFGHIJ — AL — 83210

Addison-Wesley Publishing Company
Medical/Nursing Division
2725 Sand Hill Road
Menlo Park, California 94025

PREFACE

I want to express my appreciation for the lovely farewell party. I will always have a soft place in my heart — or maybe it's in my head — for nursing.

On this note, a brilliant nurse-educator left the field for another occupation. I was sorry to see her leave, but I was not surprised. After 10 years of advising nursing students, consulting to groups of practicing nurses, and reviewing the nursing literature, I wondered only that she had remained in nursing so long (20 years), and that she was leaving ambivalently, not angrily. Anger, rampant or disguised, is nursing's hallmark, and attrition is part of its process. This is a strong statement and will undoubtedly, and rightly, be questioned.

The Nurse's Quest for a Professional Identity attempts to explain why nursing is subject to a high rate of both student and graduate attrition and why so many nurses who leave the field do so in anger. The seeds of this book were planted in 1960 when I began teaching a course in human development at several schools of nursing. I was surprised by the number of nursing students who sought me out to discuss personal and vocational problems. This did not happen when I taught the same course at local colleges. In 1969 the influx of troubled nursing students was so great that I suggested to one school director that she needed more than a counselor, which the school already had — she needed a full time psychiatric unit. She proposed instead a crisis intervention unit to provide short-term therapy to students suffering from academic or personal crisis. Since funds and professional time were severely limited, students were allowed up to eight sessions of therapy. After these sessions, the students were usually referred to other mental health facilities.

The program's extraordinary popularity with students, faculty, and hospital staff led to the project's expansion to include mandatory group therapy for underachieving students and optional group and individual consultation for the faculty (see Appendix B). The mandatory aspect of the group therapy eliminated the program's excessive popularity, but the project did cut the school's attrition rate in half.

The program was based on the assumption that student problems were psychological in nature and could therefore be mitigated by therapy. This assumption, I found, was wrong. Certainly there are students and nurses with psychological problems, but individual pathology cannot account for all the anger or troubles in nursing. (Even if this phenomenon were individually based, one might ask why nursing attracts so many troubled and angry young women.)

A review of the literature revealed two major issues that might contribute to nursing's problems: there is great dissatisfaction among nurses with their occupation (Reinkemeyer, 1968; Lewis, 1976; Fromm, 1977; Watson, 1977; Santo, 1978); and there is no consensus on the definition of the nursing role. Interestingly, despite all the changes proclaimed by the field's leaders, Reinkemeyer, in 1968, and Santo, in 1978, reported the same complaint: hospital nursing is too ritualistic and autocratic, and hospital nurses are too bureaucratic and authoritarian.

The American Nursing Association has contributed more to the issues than to their resolution. It has defined the professional nurse and the differences among the three types of educational programs (B.S.N., diploma, and A.D.) in ways neither understood by the public, accepted by deans of nursing schools (Kohnke, 1973), nor recognized by employers (Reichow and Scott, 1976). The controversy over the nurse's role is heated. Many nursing leaders express anger at attempts to protect the diploma system, which they see as preventing nursing from becoming truly professional. Diploma graduates resent the insistence on the B.S.N. degree for professional practice (Hillsmith, 1978). This fomention has not helped nursing. Many practitioners are leaving the field either because they do not like the bureaucracy and authoritarianism or because of the controversy over the nurse's role.

The Nurse's Quest for a Professional Identity focuses on the role of professional socialization in nursing. The education of nurses plays a critical role in determining nurses' reactions to bureaucracy and authoritarianism and their conception of the nursing role. Are schools and curricula organized to produce self-confident, independent, and professional nurses? Which elements in the educational system encourage or inhibit a student's professional development? Are nursing students taught to implement the modern, professional, and broad-based theories of the nursing process? In this text, the model of professional socialization is used to analyze nursing education and its role in the professionalization of nurses and to generate ideas for change in the educational system.

This book is for nursing students preparing for professional careers; nursing educators concerned about professional issues and their own role in the professionalization process; and all nurses interested in understanding the nature of nursing, identifying the roots of the problems, and recognizing opportunities for change. It is written for all who chose nursing because they believed it would allow them to be of service to others and now feel short-changed.

ACKNOWLEDGMENTS

Much of the factual material in this book was amassed during the 4-year span of the HEW grant. The theoretical scheme to explain the findings emerged upon the completion of the project when all the multiple facets had to be put in order. This project spanned many years (the original pilot project was proposed in 1969) and many people contributed to the final product.

The pilot project started at the request of Pauline Gesner (then director of Cook County School of Nursing). Her unfailing support, encouragement, and personal involvement were indispensable in setting up the project and obtaining funding from HEW. Drs. Richard Horman and Howard Rubin were my assistants at that time; devout thanks are due them for helping ride out the storms of the start-up period. During the course of the grant, Dr. Richard Smith and Mrs. Frayn Utley of the Health Hospital Governing Commission of Cook County contributed to the direction of the project.

Many assistants worked long and hard in the direct service programs and at data collection and analysis. Kathy Besser and Diane Frank taught the developmental sequence for the Pediatric Department. Active as therapists and in the data collection were Anne Brown, Richard Childs, Dr. Jim Dugo, Dr. Steve Labbie, Dr. Michael O'Mahoney, Dr. Nancy Orlinsky, Dr. Bernie Raden, and Robert Smith. Molly Brown and Agnes Tom organized special aspects of the data for their thesis. Special thanks are due to Drs. Rubin, Dugo, and Labbie who compiled the bibliography on the personality characteristics of nursing students and their relation to attrition. Thanks go to our consultant, Dr. John Sims, who always managed to bring order out of recurring chaos. The project secretaries, Mary Tirado and Kristine Hansen, valiantly labored to decipher my handwriting, to control and file a burgeoning mass of data, and to prevent the project from lapsing into chaos. They deserve not just thanks, but gratitude. When the book emerged in its present form, Juanita Pratt took over the secretarial and administrative chores. In this final phase, she, Bob Smith, and Dr. Elsa Baehr ensured that the product saw the light of day.

Thanks to the directors of diploma programs in the Chicago area who allowed us to test their students. Special thanks to all the students who participated in the extensive testing sessions.

During the course of my musings and deliberations on the problems in nursing and the professional socialization process, many people served as sounding boards for my ideas. It is a pleasure now to acknowledge their contributions, both to the substance of the manuscript and to my emotional well-being. Dr. Margery Mack and Mary Ellyn Chadwick (a director of CCSN) contributed their perception and experience. Thanks, not only for encouragement but for the time and effort they spent critiquing various drafts of the manuscript are due to Mary Daly and Ruby Mitchell (present director of CCSN). They always managed to leave me feeling that I had made progress even as they nudged me to drop the sociological jargon.

In a category of her own is Dr. Sharon Barnartt, without whose efforts and chapter revisions this project would not have reached completion. She is primarily responsible for the sociological emphasis in the manuscript and for the chapters that detail the structure and culture of nursing education and the personality variables that help or hinder progress to professionalism.

In a unique category belong Cathy Conover and Kathy Downs, who took over during the final revisions and edited, typed, and calmed me down during the final weeks. To them, as to the rest, thanks not only for the work accomplished but for their generous spirit and encouragement.

In the final category of those due thanks for patience and fortitude during this period — especially during the last year — is my family: my children, Barney and Sarah, without whom this book would have been finished earlier, but it would not have been as much fun along the way; my husband Jerry Rose, who was also my editor and severest critic — it is a tribute to his devotion that the manuscript is finished and he is still my husband; and the one enlightened reader I can always count on, my mother. Her support never faltered during the course of this or any other project I have undertaken. And thanks to my late father, who always maintained that someday I would be a doctor and an author. I wish he were here today to see his second prediction come true.

Although many people have contributed to this book and have helped to complete it, I take sole responsibility for any errors.

Helen A. Cohen, Ph.D.

CONTENTS

Part I

THE THEORY OF
PROFESSIONAL
SOCIALIZATION

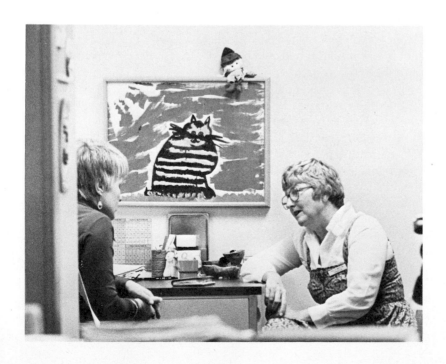

Chapter 1

INTRODUCTION

Florence Nightingale's establishment of a nursing school in conjunction with St. Thomas' Hospital in 1860 was one of the first steps in transforming nursing (at the time a rather seamy occupation) into a profession.

Society as a whole and medical technology in particular have changed dramatically since Nightingale's innovations. Nursing has been in the forefront of the improvements that have taken place in health care delivery systems. However, despite its contribution to the health care field and the ever-increasing need for nursing services, nursing has yet to take the final steps that would transform it from an occupation into a profession. Many nursing educators will take umbrage at this statement. However, a review of the nursing literature from 1969 (when H.O. Mauksch characterized nursing as "churning for change") to the present reveals the problems that nursing has had in defining itself as a true profession.

Titles of articles in recent nursing periodicals illuminate the scope of these problems: "The Nurse as Lackey: A Sociological Perspective" (Lewis, 1976); "The Need to Differentiate a Nursing Self" (Winstead-Fry, 1977); "Role Conflict in Nursing" (Watson, 1977); and "The Problem in Nursing: Nurses!" (Fromm, 1977).

Nursing remains at the stage that Simpson and Simpson (1969) classify as "semiprofessional." In a semiprofession there is a desire to provide total service without a firm theoretical base that will specify and give priorities to tasks and functions. Simms (1977) sums up the problem: "Nursing has been in the throes of seeking recognized professional status. In order to do this, nurses must prove that they have met the requirements society demands of a profession; i.e., autonomy, distinctive expertness, and control over practice and education." The nurse's "distinctive expertness" depends on a theoretical stance which delimits the profession's knowledge base.

Hassenplug, in a keynote speech at the American Nursing Association (ANA) conference in 1977, recognized the problem and recommended a massive resocialization program so that "nursing can move from its present confused, divisive state to the presentation of an effective, unified, professional front."

The question that this book addresses is: Why, after over a century of service and a decade of intense discussion of the problem of professionalism, has nursing not achieved its goal of being a full-fledged profession, with a well-defined knowledge base and a territory to call its own?

To gain perspective on the problems facing the nursing profession today, this book examines the varied experiences of nursing students as they try to integrate professional values into their self-concepts. Integration of professional values into an individual's self-concept is never an easy task. Bucher and Stelling (1977) detail the multitude of problems involved in preparing beginning professionals in any field for roles and careers that change rapidly both in values and in technology. Educating the professional nurse is an even more complex and arduous project than educating neophytes in other professions.

This book examines the role of the educational system in the socialization of nursing students and focuses on aspects of nursing education that impede professional socialization of nurses. This venture into the complex issue of nursing education undoubtedly seems presumptuous, particularly to nurses when they realize that this analysis comes from an outsider.

My colleagues and I did not start with such a grand design. Our research began with a straightforward clinical project that was designed to stop, or at least reduce, nonacademic nursing attrition. This program focused on students' emotional problems that interfered with scholastic performance. It was a long journey to the final objective. It meant traveling the intellectual pathway (which is slow, and frequently frustrating) from one set of concepts, psychological in nature (student underachievement as a neurotic emotional process), to another broader, more sociological, perspective (student failure as one part of the socialization process). Many complete revisions in both the project's theory and the service programs were necessary to arrive at the present endeavor: describing the complex process that allows the individual to become intellectually and emotionally comfortable with a professional role.

THE ORIGINAL PROJECT

The genesis of our original project lies in the work done on underachievement by Roth and others (1963, 1967, 1970). They view underachievement among college students as a neurosis derived from problems in the latency stage of childhood. In this stage, individuals learn the tools of culture (reading, writing, and mathematics) as well as attitudes toward work and toward themselves as workers. Roth and co-workers hypothesize that a primary neurotic life style problem could develop at that time, and they called this problem the "nonachievement syndrome" (NAS). An NAS student would rather fail and become childlike and dependent than renounce a comfortable life style and become independent and mature. Roth postulated that a confrontation type of group counseling, forcing the NAS student to look at the excuses given and the desire for failure, would improve both the individual and his or her grade point average. Confrontation group therapy with male engineering students verified his hypothesis (Roth and Myersberg, 1963).

Since the technique had worked so well with samples utilizing male populations, we decided to try the treatment with a predominantly female population. Surprisingly, the literature at that time showed only one study (Shaw and McCuen, 1960) on the differences in achievement between males and females, and that study merely acknowledged that there might be differences. There was no research on the treatment of female underachievers. This lack of research was surprising in view of Horner's projective study (1969), which indicated that success might be threatening to any female who was ambivalent about her own academic or professional achievement.

At the same time that my staff and I were seeking a female population to treat, the director of a local diploma school of nursing was looking for a program to stem student attrition. Historically, her school had an overall dropout rate (academic and nonacademic) averaging 50% — substantially higher than the national norm of about 33% (see Chapter 6). Intellectual inadequacy was not the reason. Based on entering academic predictive scores, all admitted students should have been able to graduate. All the failing students fit Roth's classification of underachiever; that is, students who had failing or poor grades although their scores on ability and achievement measurement tests indicated the capability to do the work.

After we analyzed five years of exit interviews, two factors emerged as significant components of attrition: emotional problems and an inability to accept the demands of the nursing role. When the school's director realized the importance of these findings, we were asked to propose and develop an attrition-prevention program for nursing students. (See Appendix B for a summary of HEW Grant Report.) The project was to be twofold: It was to focus on identifying emotional reasons for attrition; and it was to demonstrate the effectiveness of a psychologically oriented intervention package composed of confrontation group therapy, individual crisis treatment, and remediation in basic skills.

PROJECT TWO

This simple project designed to prevent attrition had to be dramatically altered when external factors shifted the philosophy of the school and the composition of students in the entering class. Just before our target population matriculated, a new administration took over the school, changing the school's organizational structure and, at least implicitly, its educational philosophy. More important to us was that drastic changes occurred in the size and composition of the target class. There were 32 more students than the originally planned 60; 38% of the class now had National League of Nursing (NLN) scores predicting certain failure.

This distortion in the student population resulted from a school-sponsored summer program aimed at recruiting students from the lower income, inner-city, Black and Latino communities. The program stressed remedial reading, writing, and mathematics for high school graduates whose basic skills were inadequate to meet entrance standards. At the end of the summer, the administration decided to admit 32 of the 45 summer students on the basis of their improvement in math and reading. It ignored their end-of-summer NLN scores, which would have made their admission to the regular nursing program unthinkable; the predicted failure rate of the 32 was 100%.

With one-third of the class marked for failure, the school did not seem to be the ideal place to run a program for underachievers. If we were to address the problems of this class, we needed to expand and change our programs and, most importantly, implement programs derived from a body of knowledge we had not investigated or even considered in our original proposal. The focus of the project shifted from the problem of underachievement to the problems of minority students in a professional nursing program. It became necessary to investigate the problems of the educationally disadvantaged with all learning processes, as well as the problems of all nursing students with the nursing educational process. The latter research led us to the conclusion that the history of nursing as a profession, its problems with a theoretical base, and the current structure and climate of opinion in nursing were contributing to the withdrawal of the students we had observed and treated.

The remainder of this chapter is an overview of some of the factors we perceive as contributing to the problem of professionalism in nursing, followed by an outline of our approach to this book.

PROBLEMS IN NURSING

The Physician as the Left Hand of God (Richman and O'Donnell, 1978)

The first problem we observe is nursing's continuing stance of submission to medical authority. Our literature review indicates that there is much controversy about whether this is so, whether it continues to be so, and what can be done about it.

Rogers (1972) ably makes a case that nursing is a profession with a defined identity and knowledge base whose function is not determined by the medical profession. Most authorities in the nursing field would probably agree that this is the ultimate goal, but many do not agree that this applies to the present status of the profession. Senior nursing students, regardless of their type of program, and graduates trying to manage a ward can attest to the fact that Rogers' view exists in theory, but not yet in fact. Nurses currently in the field and even advanced students are able to relate good examples of what Stein (1971) calls the "doctor-nurse game;" that is, a nurse subtly telling the physician what is medically correct without appearing to encroach on his authority. Thomstad and others (1975), however, think that the rules of the game have changed. The doctor-nurse game is discussed more fully in Chapter 10.

A Nurse Is A Nurse Is A . . .

A related problem, and a controversial one, is the definition of the nursing role. Rogers (1972), the ANA (1965), and Montag (1951, 1964) all maintain that there are two separate levels of nursing functions and that these levels should be taught by two separate educational systems. According to these theorists, profound differences exist between the "professional nurse," who can carry out complex functions and should be a university graduate, and the "technical nurse" with a junior college education. Complex functions are those that require a broad theoretical knowledge base: problem-solving, priority-setting, and taking responsibility for health care delivery. Technical functions are the more mechanical and concrete tasks of nursing.

Rogers (1972) disagreed completely with the idea that "a nurse is a nurse." She states: "Denials of the reality of professional and technical careers in nursing are not only fallacious, they are ridiculous." The ANA paper (1965) defined in detail the skills and attributes of the "professional" and the "technical" nurse, and since then many educators have wholeheartedly embraced Rogers' view. They maintain that there is no confusion in the definition of role or the type of education needed. However, the state of nursing education programs today does not substantiate this view.

There are three different types of nursing education programs: the diploma program, usually 3 years in a hospital-based school; the associate degree (A.D.), normally 2 years in a junior college; and the baccalaureate of science in nursing (B.S.N.), a university-based 4-year program. How does this educational system fit in the dichotomy between professional and technical? The theory does not fit reality, and for the last decade the diploma graduate has been caught in the middle as the profession has wrestled with the problem.

The controversy over the nurse's role is reflected in the ANA position papers and writings of various researchers. The ANA's 1965 position paper implies that only B.S.N. students are professionals. However, a 1973 ANA paper appears to retract this position. Or does it? Different interpretations have been advanced about the 1973 paper; some (such as Jacox, 1973) view the paper as merely a tribute to the excellent care given by diploma graduates. Other researchers have found that educators and employers see no direct correlation between any of the different educational programs and professional and technical functions (Kohnke, 1973; Reichow and Scott, 1976). The 1978 ANA conference after much debate voted to adopt *Resolution 56: Identification and Titling of Establishment of Two Categories of Nursing Practice.* This resolution calls for the two categories to be clearly identified and defined by 1980, and stipulates that the B.S.N. be the minimum preparation for entry into the profession by 1985. (The resolution concedes that implementation of these actions may be complicated by the fact that the Council of State Boards of Nursing separated from the ANA as of June 1978 and would not necessarily endorse these proposals. If they endorsed the resolution, they might not follow the same timetable.) Jacox (1978) wrote a bitter article on the problems she foresees in the twenty-first century as a result of the delays and dissention among nurses now. She feels certain that delay will mean relegation of the nursing role to the bureaucratic, nonprofessional functions. Meantime, nurses without university degrees protest having the B.S.N. forced upon them as the "professional" degree when they view themselves as competent and professional without it (Hillsmith, 1978). The controversies swirl on!

Another Significant Problem

We assumed when we began our study that the major problem in nursing was student attrition. We then found that attrition has a second victim, the licensed practitioner. That fact has gradually come into focus and greatly concerns the nursing profession. Corwin, Taves, and Haas (1961) were the first to discuss the phenomenon of fledgling nurses dropping out during the first year after graduation. They ascribe this to "professional disillusionment": students' professional values acquired during the educational process come into conflict with bureaucratic values in the work setting.

Kramer (1974) builds on Corwin's concept of professional disillusionment to explain this phenomenon and labels it "reality shock." The new graduate encounters this shock when she finds that caring for patients and assessing their needs are given lower priority than the repetitive nonjudgmental tasks forced on the new graduate by the bureaucratic system.

Curiously, the orientation of the investigators suggests that there are two different causes for the two types of attrition. Those focusing on student attrition look at the motivational conflicts that prevent students from becoming professional (psychological variables). Those focusing on licensed practitioner attrition look at the conflicts between the bureaucratic and professional ideologies (sociological variables) — or how the system causes intense frustration and drives practitioners out of the field.

As my staff and I conducted the programs and researched more of the literature, it became apparent that what we had viewed as *the* major problem was really a derivative of other more complex problems. It was difficult for us, as outsiders, to understand why "reality shock" or professional disillusionment should exist at all. Nursing education provides sufficient time and exposure to the concrete demands of the profession for the student to become accustomed to the reality of practice. It is difficult to imagine anyone spending 2 and perhaps 3 years in an institution such as a hospital without understanding its mode of operation and its regulations. If mental patients can learn the institutional norms of mental hospitals (Goffman [1959] indicates they learn quickly), why is it that intelligent would-be professionals do not learn hospital norms during their education? Why are well-trained new graduates shocked, surprised, and unable to cope with the reality of work?

At this point we saw the need for an examination of the educational process and the socialization process in nursing education. We hoped to learn how an individual internalizes the values and norms of the professional group and becomes comfortable with the occupational identity.

A Search for Roots

The cause of the high rate of attrition and the confusion over the educational system may lie in nursing's origins. Nursing became a predominantly female occupation when some women, notably Florence Nightingale and Dr. Elizabeth Blackwell, dared to reject the nineteenth-century stereotypical female role and established that women can provide health care.

One role for the nursing profession to follow was provided by Dr. Elizabeth Blackwell, who established the first school of nursing. Her concept of nursing was more medical and less military in emphasis than Nightingale's concept. However, the "Lady of the Lamp" exerted a stronger influence on the development of nursing, and that lamp has cast a long shadow.

Nightingale's influence on nursing remains strong. The nursing profession, as defined in the ANA's position paper on nursing education (1965), focuses on the strength of the Nightingale ideal and urges nurses to follow her prescriptions. The paper reminds nurses that Nightingale advocated:

> A school of nursing independent of the service agency, but providing education for service. Competent nurse-teachers and well-selected learning opportunities. The development of the student as a person. The dignity of the patient as a human being. The provision of nursing as a community service as well as for institutional care. The identification of the basis on which nursing is founded; for example, environmental hygiene and personal care. The direction of nursing by nurses. The model of the nurse as a person of culture as well as a competent practitioner.*

*From the American Nurse's Association Committee on Education, 1965. Position on education for nursing. *American Journal of Nursing* 65(Dec.):106.

Ironically, Nightingale established and promulgated an educational system that does not produce professionals like herself: staunchly independent women who discard the female stereotypes and refuse to accept the convention of traditional health care.

Bullough (1975a) discusses the contradictions and ironies in the "Nightingale Image":

> Her work as a nurse at Scutari during the Crimean War was reported in great detail by the British press and it made her a heroine to the mass of people. Unfortunately for today's nurses, however, Florence Nightingale never worked directly. She was a master manipulator who was able to get other people, usually men, to speak for her while she pretended helplessness. In Scutari, although she came with significant power delegated to her by the Secretary of War, she refused to allow the nurses under her command to give any care to the suffering men until the surgeons "ordered" them to do so. This mechanism gained her the support of the army doctors, who were very suspicious of her as well as the 38 nurses who came with her, but it also helped establish the surgeon as superior to the nurse.*

Nightingale encouraged a system that made nurses subordinate to physicians. Bullough (1975a) argues that it is an oversimplification to blame the subordination of today's nurses on Nightingale, a representative of the Victorian era. The real culprits she says, are the twentieth-century followers who have uncritically accepted the concept of subordination to the doctor.

In addition to subordination — a concept that may or may not have been accepted uncritically — Florence Nightingale established an approach to nursing education with far-reaching effects. This approach has created problems that have not yet been resolved. Her system produced practitioners who did as they were told, adding a professionally submissive role to the traditionally submissive female role. However, "professional submissiveness" is a contradiction in terms. A submissive occupation will never meet the requirements society demands of a professional occupation: autonomy, distinctive expertness, and control over practice and education (Simms, 1977).

Other Problems

What other factors have influenced the field of nursing and produced problems? Various writers suggest that problems arise because nursing is a predominantly female profession, or because it has its roots both in the military and the religious (the first school founded by Nightingale was connected with a religious order). The lack of autonomy of the nurse within the hospital is also cited, as is the confusion over the role of nursing and its lack of a definitive knowledge base of its own. These factors are discussed throughout this book as they relate to the professional socialization of nurses.

*From Bullough, B. 1975(a). Barriers to the nurse practitioner movement: Problems of women in a women's field. *International Journal of Health Services 5(2):310.*

OVERVIEW

To understand the causes of nursing student attrition we had to go beyond a model focusing on individual dynamics to investigate the process of professional socialization in nursing, particularly in the education system. In Chapter 2 we define professional socialization and describe the developmental model of professional socialization that we used in our study. With this model we were able to organize and evaluate the multitude of problems we uncovered. Our model is based upon Piaget's theory of the stages of learning, Kelman's concept of social influence (1967) and Erikson's developmental theory.

Chapter 3 defines the sociological and psychological concepts used to understand the problems in the nursing field. Chapter 4 details our hypothesis that the origin of the nursing problems previously discussed lies in the authoritarian atmosphere in nursing education and the entire health care field. This authoritarianism interferes with the process of professional socialization. Nursing students are denied the experience of a critical learning stage: resistance. This places the student and later the graduate nurse in what we term "the quest for autonomy." Students, graduates, faculty, and many administrators in nursing face this lack of autonomy almost every day. Further, this problem contributes to the confusion in defining nursing theory, establishing a knowledge base in nursing, and reforming the nursing educational system. The analysis of the educational experience is continued in Chapter 5, with emphasis on the different programs.

Chapter 6 examines psychological and personality factors in the professionalization of a typical nursing student. In Chapters 7 and 8 we inspect the problems that arise from nursing being a predominantly female profession and the problems of female ethnic minority students in nursing education.

Case studies in Chapter 9 show how individual nursing students react to and cope with specific problems in nursing education. What happens to an individual faced with the problems and emotional issues of nursing school? These studies demonstrate that intelligence is not the only factor in the successful completion of the educational program, nor is mental health. Faculty and administration provide some students with the emotional support needed to continue; other students, equally intelligent and no more disturbed but with different manifestations of their problems, are allowed to drop out. The stage analysis presented in Chapter 2 helps explain why one of the best and brightest students encounters serious problems, while another young woman, less intelligent and very neurotic (whom we designated "the universal patient" because of her proclivity for taking advantage of the crisis program no matter which therapist was on duty), graduates with flying colors.

Chapter 10 contains a review and assessment of some of the programs designed to cope with specific problems such as underachievement, reality shock, a rigidly structured curriculum, and the physician-nurse relationship. We propose in Chapter 11 some solutions based on our empirical work, our study of the literature, and our theoretical model. Our primary emphasis is on restoring autonomy to the student population—the source of future practitioners—and helping them become competent, autonomous, and truly professional.

Chapter 2

DEVELOPMENTAL SEQUENCE OF PROFESSIONAL SOCIALIZATION

All o'er the earth
Angels in white,
In sickness, age and birth
Bring light.

Healing we bring
Hope and help we bring
We of Spencer too shall bring.
These brave and shining deeds we sing—
Our sister, our Nurse.*

This song and pledge is from the "Cherry Ames" series, and most nursing schools have a similar traditional song. The legend of the "Lady with her lamp" still graces their corridors. The book jacket designed for the Cherry Ames books carries this statement aimed at the impressionable teenage reader: "It is every girl's ambition at one time or another to wear the uniform of the nurse. Many opportunities of service, or adventure, or romance, make a nurse's career a glamorous one."

Many entering students continue to view nursing as an exciting and glamorous profession that will allow them to serve humanity. Seventy-five percent of 800 freshmen nursing students tested in the Chicago area in 1971 (HEW Grant, 1975) stated that they had chosen nursing because of the opportunities it offered to meet and serve people. Other studies report similar findings (Knopf, 1975). Since the Cherry Ames ideology has had such an impact on

*From Wells, H. 1944. *Cherry Ames, Senior Nurse*, p. 210.

nursing students, it may be useful to examine the socialization process depicted in the Cherry Ames series and compare it to the experience of nursing students today.[1]

Cherry Ames arrives at nursing school holding high the Nightingale ideals of social service. Her main problem is finding time to date a handsome young man (usually a physician) while keeping up with the demanding curriculum. Less important are the clashes with bureaucratic rules that arise from her idealistic view of nursing. These problems are always resolved in the last chapter. She eventually succeeds in conquering all obstacles and becomes a successful graduate nurse exploring many specialty areas.

Cherry Ames is now outdated. (The time was World War II, and penicillin was just being discovered.) Although the more sophisticated and cynical students of today may sneer, the series is still widely read and the stereotype persists. It reflects an oversimplified and unrealistic view of the socialization process. Cherry begins her studies with all the necessary attitudes and values. She knows who she is, what her goals are, and what nursing is about; and she meets all the requirements of the educational process. She chooses nursing for the right reason and never has to change herself or her ideas. With such a well-socialized student as Cherry Ames, all the educational system has to do is provide exposure to the knowledge of the field and an opportunity to practice the skills.

If the process of education were that simple for all nursing students, the problems of nursing education would be eliminated, and the present shortage of nurses would not exist because nursing graduates would be using their education instead of leaving the field.

Deans of nursing occasionally see students who are perfectly socialized and psychologically well-integrated individuals like Cherry Ames (Dustan, 1964; Wren, 1971; HEW Grant, 1975). These students enroll with all the necessary motivations and attitudes; they lack only the technical skills and knowledge. However, while certainly these types of students are around, they are no longer in the majority.

Most students today are not prepared for the technical and emotional demands of the nursing role. Their image of the nursing profession is derived from sources such as the Cherry Ames and Sue Barton books and television shows, not from real experience. They hold the values and attitudes of the lay public rather than those of the profession.

In addition to this misconception, many nursing students are experiencing the psychological problems of adolescence. Most students in diploma and B.S.N. programs are recent high school graduates (Dustan, 1964; Wren, 1971; Richards, 1972; see also Chapter 5). Often they have not yet established their own identities or goals. They hope that nursing will lead them out of an adolescent chaos into adulthood where they may occupy a meaningful social role. Unfortunately, they cannot identify with the nursing profession because the reality of nursing does not fit their expectations. The educational process does not provide students with the professional socialization that would clarify the nursing role and allow the student to integrate an emerging self-concept with the reality of nursing.

Most students and many educators assume that the biggest problems in the educational process stem from the students' lack of technical skills and knowledge, but far more than that is needed to function in the professional setting. Students need more than an academic education—they need professional socialization.

WHAT IS PROFESSIONAL SOCIALIZATION?

Professional socialization is the complex process by which a person acquires the knowledge, skills, and sense of occupational identity that are characteristic of a member of that profession. It involves the internalization of the values and norms of the group into the person's own behavior and self-conception (Jacox, 1973). In the process a person gives up the societal and media stereotypes prevalent in our culture and adopts those held by members of that profession. The process must encourage and allow neophytes to interact successfully with the field's professionals, so they can learn how professionals feel about clients, their fellow practitioners, and the problems involved in practice. The end product of professional socialization must be a person who has both the technical competencies and the internalized values and attitudes demanded by the profession and expected by the public at large.[2]

Training for a profession is akin to the socialization of a child. One can view the child as being "in training" for adulthood. The child must learn more than the mechanical skills of walking and speaking. The child must also acquire the societal values and learn to behave appropriately within the group context. In short, the child must become a member of society and hold the cultural values and attitudes of that group. The professional training process is similar. It builds those values, attitudes, and emotional reactions required by the professional role upon a technical base.

Students in professional schools are not children but are well along the path to adulthood. They begin their education equipped with stereotypes, beliefs, expectations, and ideas about the world inside and outside of the profession. They have had other roles such as daughter, worker, girlfriend, son, boyfriend, and perhaps spouse or parent. Yet they may still be childlike in their expectations of the profession. These other beliefs, expectations, and roles must all be integrated into the students' professional identity if they are to internalize the professional role.

Professional socialization is more complex than the educational process depicted in the Cherry Ames novels. Cherry views herself as an adult and a dedicated nurse when she begins her studies. Nursing provides her with the technical knowledge necessary to implement her goals and realize her predetermined identity. For real-life students the process is rarely so simple. They must experience many changes to become competent professionals.

Professional socialization has four goals. The student must (a) learn the technology of the profession — the facts, skills and theory; (b) learn to internalize the professional culture; (c) find a personally and professionally acceptable version of the role; and (d) integrate this professional role into all the other life roles.

The first goal, learning the technology of the professional field, is the most obvious area of socialization. Clearly, students must learn the facts and the theories taught in the classroom. This is the cognitive aspect of professional socialization.

The second goal is internalizing the professional culture. This culture includes the values, norms, motivational attributes, and ethical standards held in common by other members of the profession. Students not only must know the technology and put it into practice, but they must utilize it to solve new and challenging problems. Rote knowledge of theory and facts is not enough in any profession.

For example, in the health care profession, practitioners learn to deal with culturally taboo subjects, such as nakedness and death, and to cope with the fallibility of scientific knowledge. The professional culture provides the rationale for these issues and instructions on how to deal with them. Nursing students often begin their education with negative feelings about nakedness. The professional culture specifies that it is necessary for nurses to encounter nakedness and provides reasons why the students must give up their old attitudes (the ideal of selfless service to the sick and the efficacy of scientific knowledge). It also gives them procedures on how to prepare the client and themselves for the necessary nakedness.

As well as helping practitioners deal with issues specific to their profession, the professional culture exerts control over individual practitioners by reminding them about their commonly shared ideals. An example of this can be seen in the numerous references made by health care professionals in all situations — from informal conferences to position papers — about the patients' needs having priority over all other considerations. Thus, the professional culture benefits both the individual and the profession. This culture, learned through interaction with working professionals and educators during a student's education, is the basis of professional socialization.

The third and fourth goals — finding a personally and professionally acceptable version of the professional role and integrating this professional role into all other life roles — are related to the individual's search for a unique psychological identity. Every student must learn to behave in the manner considered by all as professionally appropriate. However, in any role there is more than one acceptable way of behaving. A nurse can be gentle and soothing or brusquely efficient. A nurse can be talkative or quiet, friendly or distant, assertive or deferential. All students must find ways of behaving that are acceptable both to their instructors and to themselves. Students who cannot do this will not be able to continue working in the profession after graduation. It will either be too hard on them emotionally, or other practitioners will not find them acceptable and will make this known, limiting the professional area in which they can operate.

How does the growth and learning process in nursing education — or in any other profession — occur? How is the incapable and uncertain neophyte transformed into a competent and confident practitioner?

We propose a four-stage developmental model for professional socialization that parallels the cognitive stages of children. This model is drawn from Piaget's studies on the development of cognition in children (1928). We will also examine Kelman's theory of social influence (1967) and Erikson's theory of human development (1950) in their relation to professional socialization.

First, one note of caution: This model does not imply that the entire socialization process takes 4 years to complete or that each year corresponds to one stage of development. The timing and rate of progress through the stages depends on the specific profession and to some degree on the specific institution. Each stage may require a different amount of time, and students do not always progress through the stages in order. However, the student must experience each stage in sequence to feel comfortable in the professional role.

THE COGNITIVE STAGES

The description of cognitive changes in this section is based on the stage theory of child development of Harvey, Hunt, and Schroeder (1961), which in turn is based on Piaget's (1928) work on cognitive development. Harvey, Hunt, and Schroeder propose four stages in a child's cognitive development, ranging from concrete to abstract thought. My colleagues and I propose that a similar progression must take place in learning professional skills.

Stage I: Unilateral Dependence

In Stage I the individual places complete reliance on external controls and searches for "the one right" answer. Concepts must be accepted without question from external sources because the person lacks the necessary experience and knowledge to criticize or question. The concepts are absolute, and the individual is very sensitive to the limits set by the authorities.

Stage II: Negative/Independence

In Stage II individuals attempt to free themselves of external controls by a cognitive rebellion. Students begin questioning the data and concepts presented to them. The gospel according to the instructors is no longer totally accepted. As they question previously accepted ideas, students begin to sever their reliance on external authority for concepts and facts: to defend one's own ideas it is necessary to question other people's information. During this stage students develop the ability to question. This may cause professors some dismay, particularly if the students question too much.

Most students experience this second stage as part of a group. Feelings of discontent with professional education lead students to form groups for emotional support and to arrive at collective solutions to the problems they encounter. Olesen and Whittaker (1968) found that a norm of mediocre performance arose among nursing students, and this norm set academic standards to which all students could realistically aspire. Utilizing this norm, they managed to resist any damage to their self-concept from faculty criticism of their clinical or academic performance. Becker and others (1961) found an example of group rebellion in their study of medical students' strategies for "getting through" the first 2 years of medical school. The students felt they could not learn everything assigned to them, so they studied only the material they expected to see on an exam. They established their own criteria to select what they would study. In this case, the students' rejection of their professors' ideas was not based on knowledge of contradictory evidence or on other scientific or rational principles, but on pragmatic considerations unknown to the instructors. Khlief (1974) describes psychiatric residents who rejected attitudinal and psychological explanations of disease because of their knowledge of another system—the biological.

Interestingly, a similar situation in a nursing school had a different result. Nursing students questioned the information given them by the instructors because of their prior experience in a liberal arts college (Davis and Olesen, 1963). Instead of rebelling, the students reacted with grief. Grief and, in this case, depression, could be viewed as anger turned inward. The nursing students did not manipulate the criteria as did the medical students, nor resist as did the psychiatric residents. Rather, they became depressed when they were forced to rely on knowledge that they questioned.

Perhaps medical students and nursing students react differently in the negative/independence stage because the authoritarianism in the nursing educational system makes it dangerous to be openly defiant. Perhaps it is the result of societal tolerance of male medical students' expression of resistance and aggression, and the disapproval shown toward female nursing students who exhibit similar behavior. (These points will be elaborated upon in later chapters.)

Stage III: Dependence/Mutuality

Stage III marks the beginning of empathy and commitment to others. During this stage, opposition to facts and theories is replaced by more realistic evaluations of the environment. Students begin to think more abstractly about the material and may incorporate others' ideas into their own thoughts and judgments. Their approach becomes empirical rather than absolute. The student tests facts and ideas objectively rather than accepting them solely on the words of higher authority.

Professors generally find students in this stage most interesting to teach because the students are developing the capacity for evaluative thinking. The students have a knowledge base upon which to anchor critical thought and can relate new material to their previous knowledge base. The classroom is likely to be a stimulating and exciting place as the students think through problems and intelligently critique existing solutions.

Stage IV: Interdependence

In this stage the conflict between the need for independence and the commitment to mutuality is resolved. Mutuality and autonomy are integrated so that neither is dominant. Students gain the ability to learn from others and also to exercise independent judgment in reaching solutions. By the end of this stage the students can weigh alternative theories or concepts, resolve contradictions, and synthesize a functional set of abstract standards. These standards are flexible since they are subjected to constant empirical tests and will change as new information is received. Obviously, at this stage the student is no longer a student, but a full-fledged professional.

Reaching Stage IV is important for all professionals, but it is of paramount importance for health care professionals. Physicians, nurses, and all others involved in emergency situations must be able to make judgments quickly and be able to justify their decision. In the health care professions the knowledge base is expanding rapidly, and the amount of flexibility gained in Stage IV affects an individual's likelihood of continued success in the field. Professionals must be able to fit new discoveries into their old theories and, if necessary, change the theoretical base — or else both the theories and the profession will become obsolete.

RESOLUTION IN THE COGNITIVE STAGES

This section examines Kelman's theory of social influence and Erikson's child development theory and discusses how they relate to professional socialization. Kelman's theory helps explain the external social factors that affect an individual, and Erikson's theory reveals the internal changes that an individual experiences in the different stages.

Kelman's Theory of Social Influence

Social influence plays an important role in the professionalization process. Kelman's theory of social influence (1967) helps explain how students incorporate the values and norms of the professional culture into their self-concepts. This development is a prerequisite to Stage IV, interdependence.

Kelman postulated three steps that individuals experience in a social situation. The steps are not mutually exclusive, nor do they occur in pure and distinct forms in real-life situations, but they are identifiably different steps.

The first step in Kelman's scheme, *compliance,* occurs when an individual accepts influence from another person or group in exchange for a favorable reaction from that person or group. Individuals do not adopt the induced behavior because they believe in it, but because it is instrumental in getting something they want such as social approval or a promotion.

An extreme case of compliance is the socialization of navy recruits (Zucher, 1967). Compliance with navy regulations was enforced to such a degree that civilian identities became inoperative. The "boots" were given no choices but were forced to depend on their socializers for all their behavioral cues.

A parallel case has been noted in the professional realm. Diploma schools of nursing during the 1940s and 1950s provided a similar example of control over students' actions. They too enforced compliance (Psathas, 1968).

During the compliance stage, socializers are not only the source of behaviorial cues, but they also control the systems of rewards and punishments. If students can accept their professors as successful professional role models and accurate purveyors of the profession's norms and values, the students are relieved of the anxiety inherent in a situation that demands compliance with the professors' norms and values. If the students accept the norms and values presented by the socializers (professors) as legitimate and appropriate, they will begin to learn from the socializer what a professional is and does.

Students can easily be disillusioned if their teachers appear rejecting or do not meet their expectations. They choose their field on the basis of stereotypes that seldom provide accurate pictures of the professional role or of the educational process. Disillusionment may result if there are major discrepancies between the expectations of the students and those of the instructors. Obviously the cognitive stage of unilateral dependence is less difficult when the students want to comply with the socializing institution and can accept the faculty as appropriate role models.

Kelman's second step, *identification,* occurs when the neophyte adopts the behavior of one significant person because he or she wants to be noticed by and interact with that person. Although the student imitates with little selectivity, this does not mean complete parroting. A student's past experience may influence the initial choice of which attitudes and actions to imitate.

At this time the individual's self-concept is not at stake. New values and behaviors are simply added to the individual's previous roles rather than integrated with the individual's self-concept. With this step the student carefully chooses elements of the professional cultural role and tentatively accepts a role identity that is both personally and professionally acceptable. However, this is still a period of experimentation. The student does not accept any identity as final.

During Stage III, dependence/mutuality, the student's behavior is analogous to Kelman's second step of identification. It is during this stage that students try to come to an understanding of how they can integrate their previous roles with the professional role promulgated by the faculty and mentors in the educational institution.

Kelman's third and final step, *internalization,* occurs when individuals accept the influence because they believe in it. Professionally appropriate behavior becomes part of the self-concept and is intrinsically rewarding to the student. The student must reconcile all the various norms and values and internalize one complete set of norms and values, acceptable to both the person and the profession.

Kelman's concept of internalization parallels the fourth stage, interdependence. The internalization of the professional role causes stabilization of the self-concept without eliminating the possibility for future change. Modification in values will take place if there is a new speciality or if the work setting changes (Friedson, 1970; Bucher and Stelling, 1977), and if the person encounters new subspecialties of the profession in which new values are prominent.

Erikson's Theory of Human Development

The changes in cognitive ability and the internalization of the professional role cannot leave the overall identity of the individual unchanged. Rather, the addition of new role components, including emotional, affective, and cognitive responses, must be re-integrated into the person's overall identity. A review of Erikson's (1950) five stages of child development may help explain this aspect of the professional socialization process.

Trust vs. Mistrust   Infants must develop trust in their caretakers and must learn that the world is a benevolent place. As Erikson states in his dialogues with Evans (1967):

> The basic psychological attitude to be learned at this (first) stage is that you can trust the world in the form of your mother, that she will come back and feed you, that she will feed you the right thing in the right quantity at the right time, and that when you are uncomfortable she will make you comfortable, and so on. That there is some correspondence between your needs and your

world, this is what I mean by basic trust. But to learn to mistrust is just as important . . . Actually a certain ratio of trust and mistrust in our basic social attitudes is a critical factor. When we enter a situation we must be able to differentiate how much we can trust and how much we must mistrust, and I use mistrust in the sense of readiness for danger and anticipation of discomfort. This is a part of the animal's instinctive equipment but we must learn it in terms of our cultural universe.*

Autonomy vs. Shame and Doubt/Willpower   Erikson characterizes the second stage as a difficult human crisis:

For just when a child has learned to trust his mother and trust the world, he must become self-willed, must take chances with his trust in order to see what he, as a trustworthy individual can will. He pits his will against the will of others—even that of his protectors. We are speaking only of the rudiments of willpower at this level, and obviously not of mature willpower. Only a mature person has a willpower in the full sense, but in the early stages, something fundamental develops without which the later mature human capacity cannot develop.**

Initiative vs. Guilt/Purpose   Erikson's third stage is a locomotor-genital stage. As Erikson describes it, it is not merely the period in which children realize their sexual identity and learn about love, but children in this stage also begin to envisage goals for which their locomotion and cognition have prepared them:

The child also beings to think of being big and identifies with people whose work or whose personality he can understand and appreciate. Purpose involves this whole complex of elements. For example, when a child plays, it's not just a matter of practicing his will or practicing his ability to manipulate. He beings to have projects, as it were, it is during this period that it becomes incumbent upon the child to repress or redirect many fantasies which developed earlier in his life. He beings to learn that he must be attached to concrete things, or at least to things which can materialize.†

Industry vs. Inferiority/Competence   Erikson's fourth stage is characterized as industry versus inferiority/competence. It occurs during a period of sexual latency before puberty. Children learn the basic grammar and technology of their culture. As Erikson states:

There is an enormous curiosity during this stage of life—a wish to learn, a wish to know. Piaget's work permits us to bring the cognitive elements together with the psychosocial ones, for obviously learning is not just suppressed or displaced sexual curiosities; learning contains energy of its own which Robert White (1952) subsumes as a striving for competency. I agree with him that this is a fundamental, life-long striving, but I would think that some experiential aspects of it undergo a special crisis in the "school" age.††

*From Evans, R.I. 1967. *Dialogue with Erik Erikson,* p. 15.
**From Evans, R.I. 1967. *Dialogue with Erik Erikson,* p. 19.
†From Evans, R.I. 1967. *Dialogue with Erik Erikson,* p. 25.
††From Evans, R.I. 1967. *Dialogue with Erik Erikson,* p. 26.

Identity vs. Role Diffusion/Fidelity   The adolescent stage, identity versus role diffusion/fidelity, follows the latency period. Erikson views identity as:

> . . . an integration of all previous identifications and self-images, including the negative ones . . . During puberty and adolescence the developing individual gains some conception of where he is in this universe and that takes on fundamental meaning. This idea of a positive and negative identity is a reoccurring problem for the individual as he moves through adolescence toward maturity and old age. It re-occurs again and again throughout the life of man.*

Relationship of Cognitive Stages to Erikson's Stages

Erikson hypothesizes that the assuming of an occupational identity solidifies an individual's adult personality. Erikson's developmental model is useful in describing the emotional components in Piaget's stage theory. With these two models we can examine the relation between personality development and career choice and the professional socialization process.

What emotional issues does the student in a professional school face, and how do the emotional issues influence the cognitive stages?

Unilateral Dependence (Trust vs. Mistrust)   The entering student must trust the professional world and its practitioners. This is analogous to the feeling developed by infants for their caretakers. The student should feel that the professional world is benevolent and can be relied upon for basic information and support. Students who develop this trust will be open to new experiences and will be able to try new skills and learn from error. The professional supervisor in turn must set up appropriate limits on error to prevent any serious consequences.

The entering student brings to this educational process all the previous identities and all preconceptions of the chosen field. Since both may quickly prove unsatisfactory in providing appropriate behavior cues in the new situation, faculty must be accepted as role models. Cues provided by the faculty will structure student behavior. Students will trust the information and cues and will eventually learn to function in the professional situation only if they can identify with and trust their instructors.

Negative/Independence (Autonomy vs. Shame and Doubt/Willpower and Initiative vs. Guilt/Purpose)   In this stage, analogous to the developing child, the neophyte professional must test his or her will against that of the protectors. Students must push against and test the trusted environment to assess its limits. They must find out which role demands are inflexible and which will allow negotiations. Students do this by breaking rules and experiencing the consequences. This necessary step creates a role identity compatible

*From Evans, R.I. 1967. *Dialogue with Erik Erikson,* p. 36.

with the demands of the profession and with personal strengths and weaknesses. They learn which rules must be obeyed and which professional norms are absolute and, conversely, which rules may be bent and which norms are related to the contingencies of any situation.

In addition to experimentation, students begin trying on the new professional role to see if they can do it as well as, or even better than, their instructors. In this stage students become highly critical of their mentors. This criticism does not take the form of resistance, but is expressed when students look at their mentors' performance and say, "I can do that better."

Dependence/Mutuality (Industry vs. Inferiority/Competence)   In the industry stage, children resolve the negativism of the autonomy/willpower stage and the critical aspects of the initiative stage. They become comfortable with the skills and components in the working environment of our culture. Students in professional education are in an analogous position. They are actively learning both the technical skills and professional behavior, and must experiment with various ways of enacting the professional role. Students build self-esteem with the positive feedback received from mentors, their peer group, and clients. This feedback increases the possibility that role learning will be self-directed rather than a result of imitation or rebellion. During this stage the student tries to integrate all the previous identities into a new role identity; however, the final integration of the personality in all the old roles is not achieved until Stage IV, interdependence.

Interdependence (Identity vs. Role Diffusion/Fidelity)   At this stage cognitive and developmental theories merge. Students integrate their previous identities, the professional role demands, and their own personality traits into their self-concept to create a professional role identity. The internalization of the professional culture and the acceptance of professional peers as a significant reference group aid in this task. This professional identity helps resolve the adolescent identity crisis. Reaching this stage of identity involves integrating all the characteristics acquired in childhood and adolescent development and passing through both the cognitive stages, and the steps in Kelman's theory of social influence.

The satisfactory conclusion of this stage depends on the positive resolution of all other stages. Trust is essential for the role to be learned at all; without it, the student will be unable to accept the mentors, the professional data, or the professional world. The autonomy and initiative stages enable a student, through experimentation, to learn flexibility in the professional role. Flexibility is necessary in a field with an expanding, and indeed exploding, technology. Students must reach the industry stage to derive feelings of self-esteem from their work performance.

Reaching the cognitive stage of interdependence enables the individual to reach Erikson's stage of identity: An individual feels a sense of completeness with the realizations that the new personal identity includes all previous roles and these roles have been integrated into the new professional role.

OVERVIEW

This section examines how the cognitive stages of learning, the steps to internalization of professional values, and Erikson's developmental stages relate to the process of professional socialization.

Unilateral Dependence   Dependence is usually the easiest stage for the neophyte professional. In most professions the first year or so is spent learning the technology of the field, and practice is postponed until basic theory is learned. This is true in both medicine and baccalaureate and diploma programs in nursing education.

Students spend this stage primarily listening to lectures on basic technical material. With this format, students must passively accept material presented by instructors. Whether the students also trust their instructors, believe their presentations, and comply with instructors' demands depend in part on the personalities of the instructors. However, despite personality problems that may develop between students and the instructors, students are still dependent on instructors because, without experience, students have no real basis for questions or criticism.

Negative/Independence   Students usually find the progression from Stage I to Stage II easy. As students progress through the educational program and begin to practice some of the professional techniques and skills, they must begin to find their own way to fulfill the professional role. They also come into contact with a variety of practitioners and see how theory is translated into practice. They begin the search for those components of the professional role and culture that are compatible with their self-concepts.

Since the individual enters as an adult, having already passed through the childhood stages of trust, autonomy, and initiative, these previously acquired emotional strengths emerge as the student becomes less frightened and more confident. As they gain confidence, they begin to question knowledge and techniques and weigh the importance of theory, information, norms, and values. They begin to reject certain ways of doing things, certain manners, and certain materials. As they do this, the faculty and staff signal the neophyte what must be discarded and what must be kept, which norms are inviolate and which are flexible. Students gain a sense of what can be changed and what must remain unchanged. This process of negotiation is the core of socialization.

Even if students do not go through the negative/independence stage, they will still learn the information provided by their educational program. However, it will be a mechanical interpretation of the facts. They are programmed learners, and their previous identity has not been integrated into the professional role. Instructors and supervisors may regard this as good, but when students begin their career, this highly dependent attitude creates problems. This type of professional is not fully integrated and identified with the professional role. If a crisis arises on the job or if the professional role conflicts with other roles, these individuals will probably drop out of the field. If the individual has never resisted or experimented, but remains dependent, it is unlikely that he or she will arrive at true professionalism.

Dependence/Mutuality During Stage III, dependence/mutuality, a reversal takes place. In Stage II, the students search for ways to make the role acceptable to them. In Stage III they realize that the role must also be acceptable to other professionals and to society. They must learn role limits.

Learning these limits is what Kelman defines as identification. The emotional components of learning these role limits is exemplified in Erikson's industry stage. Here the concept of dependence/mutuality, Kelman's concept of identification, and Erikson's concept of industry all refer to the same process: An individual turns to peers, tries on the new role, examines facts and self-presentations, and decides what to reject and what to keep. This is not rote learning or emulation; the students try to reconcile their experiences and knowledge from prior stages with what they know from other roles and other times. Cognitively, they reconcile their instructors' expectations and the professional value systems with their own values and expectations. In short, they work out a compromise between the professional image relayed by their instructors and their own individuality.

Students who have gained the capacity for critical thinking during Stage II are able to do this. They have the knowledge to question what has been taught and can experiment with the values and try to discover the true meaning of any situation. For example, they can understand the consequences of centering too much attention on one patient to the neglect of other patients or paperwork.

At this stage the students seek out faculty members who share their notions of appropriate role behavior. In other words, the student attempts to find a role model compatible with both personal needs and professional demands.

Interdependence In Stage IV (interdependence), experimentation decreases; the professional role is "real." This parallels Kelman's internalization stage and Erikson's identity stage. The individuals take responsibility for their own values and actions and behave appropriately with superiors, subordinates, clients, and the public. They project an image recognizable as part of the professional role. Most importantly, the professional role becomes a part of the individual's personal identity and of all other roles and values. The individual feels confident and is comfortable in the professional role, which is no longer in conflict with other life roles or other aspects of the self-concept.

WHY IS STAGE II SO IMPORTANT?

Resistance, or in developmental theory terms, negative/independence, is a crucial element in the professional socialization process. In this stage the student's role in the process changes from passive to active, and the student offers resistance to the role demands based upon prior experience and roles. Resistance is crucial for the development of two salient aspects of professionalism: the ability to think critically and adherence to the profession.

Negative/independence is crucial to the development of the ability to think critically because a professional role involves the application of theory and knowledge to problems. It does not require rote repetition of one or many actions. Professionals must make judgments and inferences from an ever-expanding knowledge base. If students are to acquire this skill, they must learn to apply their knowledge of theory to reality, not merely parrot facts in a vacuum. They must have an opportunity to argue with their instructors and disagree with the theories presented. Without this experience students will not be able to cope with the professional field; it will have expanded beyond their scope by the time they have been practitioners for 5 to 10 years, and perhaps by the time they have graduated.

Implied in all professional education is a long-term commitment to the profession on the part of the individual. The importance of this continuity to the professional community can be inferred from the reluctance of many professional schools to admit older adults to their programs.[3] The rationale is that the return would not be high enough since it takes a great deal of energy and time to educate and socialize a professional. Therefore, professionals should be able to compensate the professional community for its investment with a long practice. Also implicit in the concept of the professional role is the assumption that the individual will devote a major portion of his or her life space as well as life span to the role, and will not give up the role easily in time of crisis.

During the negative/independence stage the student begins to personalize the professional role and internalize the concepts, and this stage determines the relationship between the professional role and the individual's identity or self-concept. An optimal fit between professional role and individual identity assures continuity in the professional role. This is what Goffman (1961b) calls "attachment to the role."

Attachment to the role is necessary for a student to learn to think critically and to have a sense of commitment to the profession — in other words, to become professional.

How do the theorists mentioned view the negative/independence stage? In Kelman's theory of social influence the internalization can only occur if the individual finds the content of the culture acceptable. This will occur if a common ground can be found between the professional culture and the idiosyncratic needs of the individual. Kelman assumes the individual will find the common ground. There is nothing in Kelman's scheme to indicate a period of active display of discontent and disillusionment. Piaget hypothesizes that this common ground can only be found if first there is a testing period. Erikson hypothesizes that to find this common ground the individual must develop autonomy and initiative, the ability to pit one's will and one's projects against those of the mentors.

FAILURE IN THE PROFESSIONAL SOCIALIZATION PROCESS

There are many paths to failure. Problems in the socialization process may occur if students skip a stage. Since stages build on each other, it is difficult for the student to resolve the next stage. For example, in the negative/independence stage, the expression of the individual's will within the constructive limits of the profession requires that the person trust the environment, its limits, and the socializers. If this trust is lacking because the individual has skipped Stage I, the experience will be total rebellion, not autonomy. The individual must learn to differentiate between autonomy — being one's self — and rebellion, refusing to do what others want. If nursing students do not trust the faculty and the information they convey, they will automatically disregard both. For example, if the faculty emphasizes neatness and cleanliness, and students do not trust the faculty, the students might rebel by appearing on the units unkempt and dirty. When this happens, not only the instructors but the entire staff becomes upset. The students feel they have exercised autonomy, but in fact it is only rebellion. As a result they become the target of much negative feedback.

Fixation is another way socialization can fail. If students become fixated in resistance and continue to be rebellious, the school will eject them or they will quit. If they do continue in the educational institution their adjustment to the mutuality of Stage III will be difficult. Their peers will probably take a dim view of their actions. They will be considered difficult by faculty, peers, and the entire health care professional community.

A third kind of failure can occur if the student is cognitively in Stage IV, interdependence, but has not reached the corresponding emotional stage (Erikson's stage of identity and Kelman's step of internalization). If students feel capable and independent as far as technical skills and intellectual understanding, but have not yet internalized the professional role, they are not yet, according to Goffman (1961b), attached to the role. The profession does not help answer the question, "Who am I?" The student must find the answer in a posteducational experience. Under these circumstances, if the first professional experience is not positive, professional attrition is likely to occur.

A blatant discrepancy between the previous identity and the professional ideal can also make the socialization process difficult. In this case, the individual may approach a schizophrenic state, having to act one way in one role and quite differently in other roles. This has been described by female physicians interviewed by Ginzburg (1966), and it certainly is not conducive to role continuation during times of stress. What has been found true of women in medical school has also been found true of ethnic and racial minority students in other professional schools (Feldbaum, 1977). As more minority students enter professional schools, there may be an increase in the number of students whose identities are far from the currently approved professional identity. Attachment for those students will become an issue particularly when role demands compete with each other. If a woman's professional role conflicts with the traditional wife/mother role, she may be forced to relinquish one role, or at least parts of the role. If attachment to the professional role is high, it will probably continue to have top priority since it provides a high level of gratification. In this case the woman might have to give up the traditional role of wife and mother. In the case of the socially mobile, it appears that identifying with a profession leads the individual to abandon the values portrayed by his or her family of origin (Handlin, 1952).

CONCLUSION

To return to our original example, Cherry Ames comes to nursing well-prepared for the socialization process. Nursing is a part of her identity, and she has no need for rebelling against the profession or resisting the rules. She depends on her peer group for social enjoyment rather than emotional or behavioral support. She worries about mastering the technical material and earning supervisors' approval. The educational process is designed to expand her knowledge, not change her behavior.

To generations of readers, this appeared to represent the epitome of nursing socialization. However, it is possible that Cherry Ames is fixated in Stage I. Perhaps she has not acquired an independent identity as a nurse or the capacity to make decisions under difficult conditions. What looks like an ideal student nurse might really be a deficient practitioner.

Cherry Ames never experiences Stage II resistance in any of the books, and the lack of a search for autonomy may mean that her identity is based upon a childlike deference to authority. Certainly her professional identity does not contain the professional attitudes and behaviors and the well-integrated identity of a decision-maker necessary for the competent practitioner.

Hott (1977), in her charming article updating Cherry Ames, presents elements of a revised version of the series for today's reader. First, she states that the book jacket would read:

It is every girl or boy's ambition at one time or another to be a nurse. One may wear a uniform or one may not. The many opportunities for service, for learning, and for independent judgment make a nurse's career an exciting one. That at least a million readers know and admire Cherry and Charles Ames, have laughed over their sense of humor in deriding the bureaucratic health care system, and have thrilled over their research projects and have wept over their experiences with death and dying. In case you have missed one of these books, here is a list of the new books in the series.*

She suggests titles such as, "Cherry and Charles on Strike," "Cherry and Charles — Consumer Advocates: They discover that when the nurse or doctor is the patient, consumer advocacy gets new blood." "We Have Met the Enemy and It Is Us, Says Cherry." Other titles might be "Carmen and Carlos, Ghetto Nurses," "Ms. and Mr. Ames, B.S., R.N.," and "Doctors Cherry and Charles Ames," where they solve the mystery of how to carry a full workload and do research at the same time. The last suggestion is "Cherry and Charles, Family Nurse Practitioners" in which "sister and brother each have competing independent practices as family nurse practitioners, further complicated by the mystery of how to secure adequate child care for their own families. A subplot involves Cherry, now a pregnant single parent and the mystery of how she will be able to practice what she preaches about family planning and family-centered care."*

Hott's article is a plea for nursing independence, asserting that nurses are beginning to assume more independent and less timid roles despite the old stereotypes, and are beginning to tell physicians when they think their diagnoses, treatments, or attitudes are wrong. She believes that nurses can attain power and effect change in the health care system. She points out that they have power in sheer numbers alone, and as the largest group of health professionals they could exercise autonomy by demanding and providing quality nursing care and assuming accountability. She concludes:

Yes, Cherry Ames is alive and well but she is changing. The traditional image is as extinct as the Cherry Ames whose nursing career would end if she married and whose school and hospital were ethnically pure. That world never really was, and the mystery is how we ever allowed nursing's image to become what it did. Let's not let it happen again.**

If Hott's recommended changes are to take place, the educational system must ensure that students are allowed to experience the four cognitive stages. Future power brokers must have experienced rebellion and resistance and learned to question authority and theory. Without experiencing all four stages, in particular the stage of negative/independence, students cannot internalize the professional role in Kelman's sense nor achieve the sense of identity

*From Hott, J.R. Updating Cherry Ames. *American Journal of Nursing* 77:1581.
**From Hott, Updating Cherry Ames, p. 1583.

described by Erikson. Without these attributes the individual lacks the emotional base necessary to take command.

Certain structures and cultures in the profession and in the educational system are necessary if the student is to go through the cognitive stages sequentially and resolve them properly. Additionally, students must have certain personality dynamics. The next chapters will discuss the social structures and cultural climate necessary for the progression to Stage IV, interdependence, and the personality characteristics that help students become independent practitioners.

NOTES

1. Cherry Ames entered into a diploma program, a population not now considered representative of nursing students in general. Our view, based upon an extensive review of the research on the sociological and psychological characteristics of nurses, indicates that the student populations in all three types of programs (B.S.N., Diploma, and A.D.) are much the same and encounter similar problems. See Chapter 5 for an extensive discussion of this point.
2. From among the many definitions of "profession" in the literature the most general were chosen to identify the many dimensions that distinguish this type of role from others. Greenwood (1972) identified five dimensions of professional roles: possession of a systematic theory, recognition by society of the profession's authority, community sanction, shared ethical codes, and possession of a culture. Goode (1972) defined the ingredients of a professional culture as a sense of identity; a systematic set of norms, values, and role definitions; a common language; and definitions of the limits of membership. Pavalko (1971) added three more dimensions: relevance to basic social values, such as health or justice; an extended training period during which the symbolic or ideational as well as the practical are emphasized; and the motivation to serve in a calling rather than (primarily) for money. Other dimensions that have been identified as distinguishing professional from other roles include autonomy, control over the knowledge base of the field, and control over working conditions (Friedson, 1970).
3. The practice of denying admission on the basis of age is on the decline. As an example, older females who have raised their families are insisting on their right to enter medical school. *Cannon vs. University of Chicago* (U.S. Supreme Court, 1979) was a recent well-publicized case. A woman surgical nurse was denied admission to medical schools solely because she was over 30 years old. The U.S. Supreme Court authorized her to sue the medical schools for the right to be considered solely on academic grounds.

Chapter 3

SOCIOLOGICAL AND PSYCHOLOGICAL FACTORS

SOCIOLOGICAL FACTORS

There are two types of sociological conditions involved in the professional socialization process: structural and cultural. Structural conditions are the underlying factors of any situation and the rules that specify interrelationships between these factors. Cultural conditions are the idea systems prevalent in society as expressed in words, symbols, and ceremonies. These words, symbols, and ceremonies are referred to as the cultural climate (Merton, 1968; Bucher and Stelling, 1977).

The structure of the sociological environment defines the series of positions, or roles, into which people fit without regard to individual characteristics. For example, the structure of the family in our society includes the positions for a father, a mother, and at least one for a child. The structure also defines prescribed relationships between these positions. In professional socialization there are positions or roles for students and mentors. There is also a situational context, which includes the place (such as classroom, laboratory, or practice location), class size, method of evaluating students, number and type of mentors, and rewards available within the system.

Structural conditions and cultural conditions interact with each other: The cultural climate arises from the structural relationships and establishes norms of behavior; these norms of behavior in turn influence the cultural climate, which then structures the relationships within the system. Thus the norms of interaction between an American father and daughter in the 1980s reflects the values placed upon children and the taboos of incest, child abuse, and infanticide (the cultural climate). A father in the typical American family would not feel that it is necessary either to marry his daughter or to sacrifice her to the gods. Indeed, there would be social and legal sanctions against this (structural conditions). In Ptolemaic Egypt, father-daughter marriage was sometimes considered necessary for the preservation of the realm; in tales of ancient Greece, sacrificing a daughter to the gods was viewed as a means of preserving the country from war. A family acting out either of these ancient norms today would be viewed as needing psychiatric treatment. In the course of history, the cultural climate has changed and has effected a change in the relationships between the structural roles.

Similarly, the professional socialization process reflects the cultural conditions—the norms and values of the professional culture that arise from structural conditions. The structural conditions are those specific educational experiences defined by the profession as prerequisites to joining the professional community. The cultural climate of the profession prescribes behavior norms and attitudes for both students and practitioners and may include overt and covert expectations of whether each group actually will achieve the prescribed norms.

The structure of the socialization process produces the observable behavior of the student; the cultural climate determines how the student feels about the behavior demanded. For example, authoritarian climates usually lead to student anger.[1] The student will express anger covertly or overtly depending upon structural conditions and how much anger he or she is permitted to display. In a permissive climate, students will feel less anger but may express their anger more overtly.

These structural and cultural conditions affect a student's progress through the cognitive socialization stages in two ways. First, they govern the ease of transition from one stage to another. Second, they determine the manner in which the transitions from one stage to another may come about. When the social structures are appropriate and the cultural climate is benign, people resolve the issues of each stage and move easily to the next stage. If problems exist in either the structure or the cultural climate, students may pass through the stages without resolving the issues of each stage. If progress is made without resolving the specific issues, the socialization process is hindered and ultimately the entire profession will suffer.

Let us first examine the structures and cultural climates that would facilitate a student's passage through the cognitive stages outlined in Chapter 2.

Structural and Cultural Conditions in the Cognitive Stages

Stage I: Dependence In cognitive theory, at the dependence stage the theoretical and factual basis of the professional field must be accepted on faith. The neophyte, lacking any other frame of reference (except possibly glamorized or comic stereotypes picked up from the media), must rely on the knowledge of the instructors and mentors.

Several structural conditions can help insure that the student progresses easily through this first stage of dependence. First, the entire curriculum outline must be familiar and make sense to the student. The student must realize the relationship between the knowledge presented in beginning courses and the usefulness of this knowledge to professional practice. Second, the mentors must present themselves as knowledgeable people worthy of trust. Students must believe that the knowledge portrayed by the faculty is trustworthy, and that the instructors are good individuals to whom the students can relate.

One structural condition that greatly helps the student resolve the issue of dependence in this first stage is variety among instructors and practitioners. With a variety of mentors the student is assured that there are many roads to competence, and that the subject matter—while occasionally difficult or mystifying—is comprehensible. A structure with variety usually gives rise to a benign cultural climate, or at least one that is not rigid in its demands. Each student will find at least one instructor or mentor that he or she can feel at ease with and trust.

Stage II: Negative/Independence   During this critical cognitive stage, negative/independence, students start to test the limits of the professional environment. They discover new behavior patterns that must be exhibited and old behaviors that must be revised or ignored.

This is a difficult time for faculty and mentors. Anyone responsible for educating the young professional must be willing to permit student resistance, even if this produces some unpleasant interpersonal encounters. They must do this not only for the sake of the student but for the profession and ultimately for themselves. At this stage students may develop the leadership traits so admired in professional circles. Students who have been able to resist the robot interpretation of the role and facts, and who have been allowed to be critical of the field and its practitioners will be able to analyze the new and different professional problems continually arising in a changing field.

The educational structure must allow students to question, resist, and test the material presented. It must provide a cultural climate that allows students to express their questioning and resistance freely without fear of reprisal. The educational structure most likely to facilitate passage through this trying stage is one that encourages the formation of student groups.

Structurally, student groups are important because they produce a student culture with its own norms and values. When students voice their opinions to their peers, their peers listen. Student leaders can emerge to serve as spokespersons for the more timid members, and conversely, timid members can provide support for the group's spokespersons. The extremely angry will be balanced by the more moderate and cautious. The group will support those students criticized by faculty. Within the group the students can sort out the relevant from what they consider irrelevant criticisms and help each student maintain self-esteem.

Since in most professional education this stage of negative/independence is concurrent with the beginning of the apprenticeship experience, feedback and constructive criticism by faculty and practitioners is necessary for good professional habits. However, this feedback may be hard on the individual's ego. Peer groups provide positive feedback to bolster the person's feelings of self-worth and help to offset the faculty's criticism of the professional behavior.

An example of peer support helping students cope with faculty criticism and with their need to resist faculty evaluation is illustrated in the case of one young nursing student who cried every time she saw a patient in pain and whenever there were staff problems on a unit. Her instructors were concerned about this "unprofessional behavior" when she was on the regular medical wards. When she entered her rotations for trauma and the intensive care unit, the instructors' concern turned to alarm. They considered her behavior unacceptable, and the administration recommended that she be suspended for unprofessional behavior. They did not believe that she could ever stand the trials and tribulations of nursing. Her friends, realizing that these emotional reactions could result in dismissal, resorted to clowning and tricks to produce laughter in tense situations. They also forcibly marched her off to the psychologist's office. She and her friends, with the aid of a psychologist, formed a group and discussed their resistance to the faculty's view that crying or showing emotion about a patient's problem was not within the scope of professional behavior.

The protection the group offered this student during her first 6 months of clinical training enabled her to finish the program. She has since progressed to professional distinction but is still critical of the notion that a professional attitude precludes becoming involved with the patient. Because of this she is frequently viewed as deviant within her nursing group, but she gives excellent technical care and is known as "the nut who cares."

The idea that student groups resist faculty and mentors may sound like war — and in some ways negative/independence parallels this conflict, much as the 2- to 5-year-old rebellion may look like war to the parents living through it. However, just as war with parents is necessary to produce independent individuals, war with the faculty and practitioners is necessary to produce independent professionals.

The group structure helps both faculty and students weather this stage. The students gain strength in numbers and the faculty finds it easier to work with a few spokespersons rather than face an entire angry class. Further, if the faculty co-opts student leaders by giving them a voice in decision-making, the faculty will appear to be on the students' side, which may diminish the strength of the resistance.

The cultural climate most appropriate for this stage encourages students to question not only the theories and facts of the profession but the professional cultural and values as well. As with the structural conditions necessary to resolve Stage I, diversity among the faculty will also help in Stage II. With diverse viewpoints it is unlikely that the faculty will be viewed as a monolithic unit demanding conformity.

Educational structures that interfere with smooth progress through this stage are programs and curricula that preclude peer group formation and the development of a student culture. If the group form of resistance cannot take place, it is difficult for an individual to display resistance. The issues of this stage cannot be easily resolved. If the cultural climate is authoritarian and questioning is discouraged, and if obedience to prescribed behavior and values are demanded, the student culture will be stifled. Progress through this stage will be very difficult.

Stage III: Independence/Mutuality   Students in the third stage, independence/mutuality, must learn the limits of the role, how to distinguish the most important information, how to set priorities, and how to maintain a professional facade. In a given situation, the students must be able to select relevant information, fit the information into a theoretical framework, make a prediction, and take action based on that prediction. These skills cannot be learned from reading a book any more than riding a bicycle can be learned from a book. Opportunities must be provided for the students to test their knowledge and analytical skills by making decisions about actual problems.

The structural conditions that best facilitate transition through this third stage is a group apprenticeship system. The apprenticeship, or clinical experience, provides the students with the necessary arena in which to try out decision-making as if they were full-fledged professionals. With instructors acting as safeguards, students can make mistakes and learn from them without jeopardizing the health or welfare of their clients.

A group apprenticeship provides the student with a support system that enables the individual to try on different types of professional roles. Students can evaluate different types of procedures with their classmates without feeling that they are being scrutinized or graded or that their passage through the school system is jeopardized because of faculty disapproval. During this stage, the individual needs what Merton (1968) has labeled "anticipatory socialization." Anticipatory socialization occurs when individuals who wish to assume a new status begin to acquire the necessary behavioral characteristics, attitudes, and role orientations prior to formally making the change. If the student behaves professionally prematurely, the faculty may consider this presumptuous. The peer group can point out problems, pitfalls, and unacceptable attitudes much more gently and without endangering their apprenticeships.

The cultural climate that promotes smooth passage through this stage encourages the students to work independently, to validate responses with their peers, and to use the faculty as a resource. The faculty should make it clear that they expect good performances from the students, and there should be an understanding on the part of both the students and faculty that the students will begin to take responsibility for themselves. As students' skills and technique increase and their knowledge base expands, they will take more responsibility and turn less to the instructors for guidance.

Stage IV: Interdependence   In this stage the conflict between the need for independence and the commitment to mutuality is resolved. The student takes leave of the student role forever and accepts responsibility for her or his decisions and actions. The apprenticeship ends and the evaluations now come from clients and colleagues. These evaluations will be indirect, unlike the direct supervision a student receives. A displeased client may sue, simply not come back, or vent his or her displeasure in minor complaints or failure to follow directions. It is sometimes difficult for the new professional to understand the workings of these subtle mechanisms of professional control after being accustomed to the direct control of the apprenticeship system.

Peer control is now subtle. Indeed, most peer control arises from the referral system (Hall, 1946). Professions do have formal structures to control the practitioner, such as tissue committees in hospitals, promotion and tenure committees in universities, professional organizations empowered to disbar, and state licensing procedures. These mechanisms, however, are not part of the day-to-day experience of the professional. Individuals must now rely on themselves to define the professional role.

Structural and Cultural Conditions in the Social Sphere

The structures and the cultural components that support progress in the cognitive stages also support progress in terms of Kelman's (1967) model of social influence in the professionalization process.

According to Kelman, the first stage (compliance) occurs when an individual accepts influence from another person or group because he or she wants to receive a favorable reaction from them. This type of behavior is encouraged by those institutions whose curriculum is well-defined, where students have a clear-cut future goal, and where the path from the entrance to that future goal is well-defined. A variety among the practitioners means that each student can find at least one or two instructors to trust, and this also facilitates the resolution of issues at this stage.

Kelman's steps to professionalization do not include the stage of resistance. We believe that the experience of resistance is essential to the socialization process. If there is no tolerance for individuality and students are given no freedom to think and act unhindered by any faculty expectations, there will be no progress within the profession. Without the experience of resistance, students may well become clones of the practitioners who are teaching them, replicating their predecessors' issues and solutions. Since most professional fields are experiencing an explosion of technology and rapidly changing demands on the professional role, if students are mere replicas of their mentors they are in effect dinosaurs, unable to adapt to the changing social climate.

According to Kelman, identification occurs when an individual adopts attitudes or behavior to please a mentor because the individual wishes to be perceived as the same type of person or as belonging to the mentor's group. The individual imitates the mentor in a selective way, utilizing those behaviors that will enable him or her to perform the professional role in an approved fashion. The behaviors chosen for emulation are added onto the individual's self-concept, not integrated into the core of his or her identity. An example is the difference between saying "I'm taking a course in biology and trying to think scientifically" and saying "I'm a biologist involved in scientific inquiry."

Kelman's identification corresponds to Stage III (dependence/mutuality), and in interactional terms this refers to students learning to play the professional role.

As with the cognitive stages, groups and the apprenticeship system are important structural components that allow the process of identification to take place. Within the group students can pretend to be professionals and test out values, personality characteristics, and self-presentation on a "live audience." Students can try out many different behavior patterns before arriving at those acceptable to themselves and the professional culture. Since the goal of this stage is finding components of the professional role that are both personally and professionally acceptable, both the apprenticeship experience (which allows the student freedom to experiment without risk of serious consequences) and a group experience (which allows the student to turn to peers for support and reinforcement) are necessary.

The cultural climate, as with the cognitive stages, should be one of trusting tolerance. Students need feedback that corrects behavior without devastating their self-image. The individual can best judge whether the values in the self-presentation are personally acceptable, but the instructors and clients must judge whether the behavior is professionally acceptable. Since the presentation of self is a sensitive area for every individual—and particularly those in the process of becoming professional—it is obviously important that the climate support the student's prerogative to experiment with different forms of role enactment.

The situation is analogous to a theatrical company that opens in New Haven preparing for Broadway. The play and the acting may be essentially good, but alterations are still necessary. Different parts or aspects of the play will be cut or expanded and different emphases may be stressed before the play officially opens. The aspiring professional will also be playing out a role—in this case a lifetime career role. This third stage of identification, or in Piaget's terms, "mutuality," provides the out-of-town tryout period where revisions can be made without closing down the production. If student groups are too large or nonexistent, this stage is not given adequate room for expression. Students will feel alienated and lost regardless of the value and quality of their work.

An example of this type of alienation occurred when a nursing school changed its educational structure to an "open curriculum," which permitted students to take courses at their own speeds. The structure was designed to foster autonomy among the students and did so, but since the students could progress at their own pace, they did not form groups. The result was a lack of student culture and a feeling on the part of the students that they were alone and burdened. They could not specifically define the burden but reported feeling "burnt out" at the beginning of the senior year. They had no group support as they tried to integrate the professional nursing role with their own personal characteristics, so they tried to act professional at all times. This is a heavy burden for the preprofessional. Ironically, the more the faculty did for the students the more the students complained that they were receiving too little time and attention from the faculty. It seems that peers are vital to this stage and feedback from faculty alone will not suffice. As one student stated, "I always feel I'm doing my damndest to put on a good show but no one comes to see it or cares."

An apprenticeship experience usually guarantees feedback from faculty. This feedback is necessary to prevent students from endangering clients and to shape their behavior into the professional mold. The fact that supervision must not be left to chance but must be structured into the system is taken for granted in the health care and related service fields. However, interaction with peers is an equally valuable but often overlooked experience.

Kelman's final step of social influence is internalization. For the professional, it is the internalization of the professional norms and values into the individual's self-concept. Kelman states, "The internalized behavior is intrinsically rewarding; both behavior and rewards gradually become independent of any external source."

The structural and cultural conditions in the socialization process are illustrated by the analysis of medical education in Appendix A. Medical education provides a good example of how structural and cultural systems provide support for the cognitive stage model and the social influence model of professional socialization.

PSYCHOLOGICAL FACTORS
AFFECTING PROFESSIONAL SOCIALIZATION

The sociological factors of structure and culture determine the progress of the average student. Personal characteristics, however, also affect the socialization process, and no student is truly "average." Educational systems with appropriate structures and a benign cultural climate nevertheless experience student attrition and produce graduates who have not internalized the professional role. Conversely, students survive and succeed in schools where the structure and climate are so psychologically punitive that the educational process resembles a mine field. This section examines those psychological factors that accelerate or inhibit progress toward professionalism.

Academic Ability

Faculty, students, society-at-large, and we (despite our personal experiences and research indicating the contrary) generally assume that academic ability is necessary for professional success. However, research on attrition in nursing education reveals that many students who score high on academic predictor tests drop out, while others with minimal scores graduate (Teal and Fabrizio, 1961; Taylor and others, 1966; HEW Grant, 1975). Why is this so?

One reason is that the tests are far from fool-proof. They measure attributes and aspects correlated with success and intelligence but cannot measure intelligence directly. Another explanation is a possible disparity between cognitive ability and psychological maturity. Social and emotional development does not always follow the same pace as the development of academic acumen. Faculty and practitioners emphasize to new nursing students the importance of independence and professional attitudes. Some very bright students live up to these expectations cognitively, but cannot integrate their cognitive knowledge into their self-concept and cannot accept the role emotionally.

One point that often bothers the cognitively mature yet psychologically immature students is their mentors' definition of the "professional attitude." Faculty, administration, and practitioners believe they are teaching students to be objective when they warn them not to become overly involved with the patient. They do this because they believe (and know from experience) that overinvolvement hampers utilization of technical skills and abilities. Students sometimes interpret this message to mean: "Be less human—do not admit your feelings." When a student leaves the program after hearing this message (and they usually do), faculty members express great regret. They wish the student had stayed a little longer so that the problem—fear, apprehension, or anger— could have been resolved.

The faculty does not realize that time can not cure this problem. Students intellectually capable of making a mature and skillful decision but lacking the self-esteem and initiative necessary to put the decision into action frequently rely upon patient feedback to develop their own self-confidence. When this is the case, the faculty's admonition about overinvolvement creates a serious conflict for the student.

This conflict is demonstrated by one nursing student who became extremely agitated whenever there was a patient crisis. She cried when her patients were in pain and became depressed when one of her patients died. Her instructor remonstrated, pointing out that such behavior was unprofessional. The student interpreted the instructor's message (helping patient requires self-control) as a demand to be less human. Predictably, since this conflict was not resolved, she dropped out of school. The problem is so common in nursing that a nomenclature and a field of research have been developed, nonacademic attrition (Teal and Fabrizio, 1961; Taylor, 1966; Cohen and Gesner, 1972), to study the phenomenon of cognitively competent students leaving school for emotional reasons.

The converse problem is one in which students learn the professional culture but lack technical skills. Usually these students have worked in a health care setting prior to entering nursing education. In their prior work situation they were treated as part of the health care team. They are not, as Kelman would put it, at the compliance step upon entering; they have already identified with the professional image. They consider themselves competent and knowledgeable and they project this image to faculty and clients alike.

This interferes cognitively with Stage I, dependency. The faculty tends to accept the mature self-presentation until the student is on the wards, where the technical skills and cognitive competency must be monitored. These students readily move to negative-independence without having resolved dependency. They resent the reviewers and feel the faculty is picking on them.

One student who skipped the cognitive stage of dependency upset not only her unit but the hospital and the entire school. This student was well-known for her maturity and ability to interact with patients in a professional manner. Her mode of presentation allowed the faculty to ignore the fact that she sometimes did not have a good grasp of the data base. When she entered her intensive care experience, the discrepancy between her cognitive development and social maturity leapt into focus. She insisted that her care of patients was better than the head nurse's. She supported this contention by pointing out that she could talk to her patients, explore their emotional problems, and make them more comfortable with their treatment. However, she ignored the fact that in intensive care the majority of patients are unconscious! These patients depend on the nurse's knowledge of life support equipment — emotional care is not a top priority.

Motivation

Another psychological determinant is motivation, or goal-directed behavior. In this context, a student's goal is professional licensure. A determined student can quickly pass through the cognitive stages, resolve the issues of these stages, and become a licensed professional.

However, motivation can also limit the individual's capacity to deal with the reality of working in a professional world. This can occur if the student prefers speed to thoroughness and passes through the stages without resolving the issues of each stage. If students are in a hurry to adopt the professional demeanor and skip the cognitive stages of negative-independence or mutuality, they lose the opportunity to integrate into the professional peer group and to modify misconceptions of nursing stereotypes. An older nursing student surrounded by recent high school graduates may have this problem. She already has a psychological identity and has started the process of incorporating the nursing role into her self-concept. She wishes to acquire the skills and knowledge to complete the process quickly. As a result, she may feel isolated from peers and faculty — by skipping the resistance stage, she does not learn to criticize the field and may not be able to accept future roles changes.

Conversely, while some students skip Stage II, many students become entrapped in this stage and the accompanying griping, resisting, and challenging. They become critics of the field and the educational institution at the expense of developing a professional identity. These students frequently emerge from the educational experience as critical as when they entered the resistance stage. They become the ''young Turks'' and launch campaigns to save the field. If their efforts to save the field prove too frustrating, they leave the field and may start in another.

The outcome for the determined tunnel-vision student who has skipped the resistance stage is largely determined by other personality characteristics and by the environment in which he or she works. The outcome for the student entrenched in the negative/independence stage is largely determined by the personality traits of the faculty. If faculty members listen with understanding to the students' dilemma and are able to demonstrate alternative ways to play out the professional role, students may find it easier to fit their particular personalities into their conception of the professional role. If, on the other hand, the faculty views any resistant behavior with horror and feels that such attitudes are unbecoming to a professional, the student is likely to leave the field.

Latent Identities

Another set of personality traits can be summed up in the concept of latent identities. Becker and Geer (1961) utilized Gouldner's (1957) concept of latent identity to explain how roles that may not appear in one situation may nevertheless influence what happens in the role currently being played. They explain:

> Gouldner's paper on latent social roles makes a distinction that is both long-needed and provocative. He distinguishes those social roles related to identities which the group agrees are relevant to a particular social setting from those related to identities conventionally defined as being irrelevant, inappropriate to consider, or illegitimate to take into account in the same context. The latter

he terms latent as distinguished from manifest, roles and identities. His research indicates that latent roles can be empirically distinguished and that they have important consequences with behavior of people in organizations. Although latent identities appears to be a sociological concept it is used here to explain personality and the interaction of personality of the professional role. All adults have latent identities which stem from religion, ethnicity, family, and form the underlying strata of the personality which shapes the way the individual plays the professional role even though these previous identities may appear to be irrelevant to the new role.*

Becker and Geer use social class as an example of latent identities that affect work behavior:

> For instance, an occupational group drawn largely from one social class will have an occupational culture dictated by social class premises more than one which draws from all levels of the class system. We might expect the occupational culture of bankers to reflect upper-middle or upper class cultures and that of steel workers to reflect lower or lower-middle class culture. While that of jazz musicians, who are recruited from all class levels, would not reflect the culture of any particular class stratum. The latent culture would restrict solutions to immediate occupation problems within the framework of the given class culture; other solutions would not occur to members of the occupation who would be rejected as illegitimate or improper. Both bankers and musicians, let us say, may find their clients or customers difficult. The musicians' solution to this particular problem—open hostility—might not be available to the bankers because of the restrictions on such behavior in their social class culture.*

An individual's latent identity may also contain such personal characteristics as aggressiveness, tolerance, and empathy. The value structure of the individual as expressed in political or religious idealogy is another source of the latent identity. All these factors—political attitudes, religious beliefs, ethnicity, sex, family role, social class—can influence the way a professional reacts to any issue. For example, religion might appear to be irrelevant to becoming a physician or a nurse, but in fact it does influence many individuals' reactions to the health care issue of abortion. Despite the changes in the health care field's professional ideology and in societal norms, the latent religious identities of many health care professionals continue to cause abortions to be prohibited in many hospitals.

Latent Identities and Professional Socialization: The Fit Between Self and Role   The presence and potency of all these latent identities are primary reasons for the difference between adult socialization and childhood socialization.

When children enter nursery school, they do not have to fit this new role—nursery school student—into an identity previously crowded with values, beliefs, and other roles. Indeed, the primary role of child is still salient

---

*From Becker, H., and Geer, B. 1961. Latent culture: A Note on the theory of latent social roles. *Administrative Science Quarterly* 5:304, 308.

within the nursery school. However, when an adult enters professional school, the desired new role must be made to fit with a constellation of roles and personality characteristics already established. How does the professional role fit in with all previous roles? Which personality characteristics enhance the role integration and which conflict with the role demands?

Becker and Geer (1961) state that "a harmonious identity role fit happens when entering individuals are junior versions of the practitioners who will become their mentors." In other words, practitioners respond most kindly to students most like themselves; conversely, the students are most likely to trust professors whose demands coincide with their own value systems.

The health care field illustrates the problems that can result when this good fit is no longer the case. In the past, professional schools tended to admit those students most resembling members of the admissions committee. The prototypical entering medical student prior to 1964 was a white male with stereotypical male personality characteristics. Cherry Ames was a junior version of the faculty that educated her. (As recently as 1968, Psathas found that nursing students who demanded more autonomy than the faculty was willing to permit — in other words, students who had deviant latent identities — were forced out of their nursing education.) Today the health field has changed, and individuals with far different backgrounds and therefore different latent identities are entering medical school and nursing. The professional socialization process is no longer as simple as it was in the past.

Let us examine the stages of professional socialization to see how a poor fit between the individual's latent identities and the values of the professional role interferes with the socialization process.

Latent identities may interfere with the first cognitive stage of dependency, Kelman's compliance step, and Erikson's trust stage. Cognitive dependence and compliance may be difficult because the student sees the instructor as an individual unlike the self, and therefore cannot imagine following in the same path or footsteps. It is also more difficult to establish mutual trust. Faculty members view these students as unlikely future professionals because they are so unlike the faculty; students think the faculty is incapable of understanding their problems because they are so different from the students. A female in a traditionally male profession or a male in a traditionally female profession are recognizable mismatches. For example, female medical students complain that they receive less support and respect from their instructors and from the rest of the staff, and that they are likely to be viewed with suspicion by patients who believe they are nurses, not physicians. Instructors in nursing schools tend to wonder why the males chose nursing; the male students tend to feel that the faculty is scrutinizing them more closely and critically than they do the female classmates (Barnartt, 1976; HEW Report, 1975).

Difficulty with dependence, compliance, and trust may push the individual prematurely into negative/independence or into Erikson's developmental stage of autonomy. Students whose latent identities are different from those of the professional group, and who act out their discomfort with dependence in their rebellion, may be excluded from the dominant student culture and labeled troublemakers by both peers and faculty. Frequently, these individuals are forced from the field. The faculty considers this necessary because the individuals were unable to fit the mold associated with the professional role.

An example of how differences in latent identities can affect the educational process was exemplified in the reactions of the black and white group of student nurses to a mass tutorial program in a diploma school of nursing. All the students appeared to be having difficulty with the basic sciences because of math deficiencies, so a special math tutorial was offered to all students. The administration posted the classes and offered the math tutorial to anyone who wished to take advantage of it but insisted that all those students who had received a grade of C or lower on the midterm examination in any of the science classes take the math tutorial course.

The black students who were doing poorly in science considered the tutorial program to be harassment. They thought that utilizing the help would mean admitting that they were stupid and did not know math—in other words, they thought they would lose face. The white students did not take the same view; they viewed the tutorial program simply as a means to pass a course. They did not consider it a comment on their intelligence. As a result, the math tutorial was attended predominantly by white students, and even those black students required by the administration to attend frequently failed to do so. As a result, most of the white students passed the basic science courses and many of the black students failed.

When the grades came in, the faculty thought the black students were lazy and did not belong in nursing—otherwise, they asserted, the black students would have attended the tutorial sessions and passed the course. The black students viewed their own failure as evidence of the faculty's racial prejudice. This conclusion was based on their interpretation of the facts: first, the faculty announced that they were dumb and insisted upon their taking a tutorial course, and second, the faculty had deliberately set the standards so high that they could flunk the black students. After all, as the Black Student Association pointed out in a petition to the school's board, it was mainly black students flunking the course; most white students passed. To them, the fact that the white students had passed and black students had failed was proof of racism.

The few hardy black students who survived this period were determined to become nurses at all costs. Indeed, some of them did take advantage of the math tutorial program, albeit surreptitiously. Most of them claimed time conflicts and tried to make sure that their peer group would not be aware they were receiving tutoring. (As discussed at the end of this section, the differences between the black students and the white students may in fact be due to differences in social class, not race. Whatever the cause, the latent identities were different, and the point here is that this difference caused these students to fail their courses.)

The cognitive negative/independence, or rebellion in Erikson's autonomy stage, comes easily to students with different latent identities. The mutuality of the cognitive Stage III and the industry and interaction with peers in Erikson's Stage IV is the most difficult for these students. First, it is difficult for them to find a group in which they can try on the professional role for size and fit. Second, if few of the values presented are acceptable to the individual, or conversely, if few of the individuals' attributes are compatible with the faculty's presentations of the professional role, the individual must seek new and untried solutions. This may involve giving up elements of their own identities, changing deeply held values, or finding a new way to enact the professional role.

In any case it is difficult to progress through the educational system without guidance from the faculty or practitioners. Every play needs a director — veteran actors can sometimes direct their own shows but neophytes cannot. The cognitive Stage IV, interdependence, Kelman's concept of internalization, and Erikson's identity stage build upon the previous stages, so it is unlikely that students with latent identities so different from the professionals would completely internalize the field's accepted values, norms, or self-presentations. Time and exposure to a variety of professional situations are needed for the individual to find unique solutions to the role and value conflict. When this conflict is intense, one of two things happen: Either the professional role is valued to the exclusion of everything else (a female physician may present an even more masculine and rigid image than her male peers [Israel and Sjorstrad, 1968]); or the individual may shed the professional role. Women who drop out of a profession to raise children do so because they believe that their children come first. They elevate the latent role of female and mother above the professional one.

Conflicts between latent identities and the professional role create problems for the neophyte that make it very difficult to resolve the issues in the stages of professional socialization. The remainder of this section discusses some types of latent identities that cause problems: sex, age, and social class.

Many investigators (Epstein, 1970; Campbell, 1971; Rosen, 1973; Barnartt, 1976) have investigated the various problems confronting the woman who wishes to become a physician. The female has been prepared by previous socialization to be unassertive and has been allowed to be emotional. This leaves her unprepared for the assertive and dispassionate role promoted by the medical field.

Males in nursing frequently report the same problems as females in medical schools (HEW Grant, 1975). Many male students complain that their head nurses distrust them and believe they are usurping a role that does not belong to them—the status of physicians. They find that as men they have more in common with the male physicians than they do with their peers, who tend to be female. They also find that many people assume that they are homosexual. Nursing is generally considered a female function and the public questions how a male can be a nurse.

The female, because of her latent identities, must be more determined to become a physician and change her values decidedly to play the role; but the male nurse, once he is graduated, does not have the same problem. He is assumed to be assertive, professional, and competent; hence he is most likely to go into administration and indeed be promoted before and beyond his female peers. (Notter and Spalding [1976] found that although males represent only 1.4% of the total nursing population, 8.2% of male nurses are top-level administrators with salaried jobs, compared to 3.8% for all registered nurses.)

Age, socioeconomic class, race, and ethnicity are other differences that can contribute to a self-role conflict. An individual's age often determines the degree of respect, deference, and authority he or she expects. The student role is inherently a nonauthoritative one, and the older student, accustomed to deference because of the age role, may feel resentful if the faculty does not show this respect. Many older nursing students complain bitterly that the faculty treats them like babies (HEW Grant, 1975). Faculty in turn complain that older students tend to be rigid and do not respond to feedback.

Social class influences an individual's time perspective and ability to delay present desire for future gratification. This aspect of latent identity also affects the individual's ability to accept the values of the profession (Miller, 1977; Handlin, 1952).

Professional education is based upon the individual's willingness to spend a number of adult years in a student role, essentially adolescent in character, with limited control over his or her environment. Middle class students have already learned delay earning of a living and taking on adult control of their lives. Lower class students, more directly involved in the frustrations of satisfying basic needs, have difficulty in delaying gratification. This too can interfere with the socialization process (Handlin, 1952). An inability to delay for future gratification can interfere with cognitive dependence, Kelman's concept of compliance, and Erikson's concept of trust. The individual cannot understand why so many demands are being made and does not perceive the future rewards. There appear to be no appropriate or approachable role models to emulate and no understanding peers with whom to identify. If these individuals are to reach the cognitive stage of interdependence, achieve internalization of the professional role, or reach professional identity, they will be forced to modify many of their traits derived from this previous social class role. They will have to lengthen their time perspective and discipline themselves to await future gratification. In so doing, they identify with the middle class and reject their backgrounds. (It is no wonder that Handlin [1952] describes the process of professional socialization for the sons of immigrants as "the path away from home.") Few professionals are comfortable in the lower class milieu, even if that was their point of origin.

The problems related to race and ethnicity are usually social class problems. Neither race nor ethnicity necessarily involve inherent role traits that impede professional socialization, but frequently the racial and ethnic students recruited for professional schools come from the lower classes. Individuals who have the middle class ethos (respect to work and deferment for future gratification) proceed to the stages of socialization with the peer group regardless of race. They may have inner feelings of alienation and wish for role models from their own race or ethnic group, but they progress through the stages in step with the rest of the class.

The example of the black students in the diploma school of nursing where there were mammoth problems with the math tutorial program illustrates this point. Both groups of students had the same values: they both believed in the profession of nursing and valued the opportunity to become a nurse. In this case, although the racial values were much the same, the differences in values between the middle-class and lower-class population were striking. The black students had been drawn from a lower-class population, the white students from a middle-class population. Therefore their presentation of self — the manner in which each group handled their aggressions, managed their time, dressed, and spoke, and the kind of image they wanted to present — created highly apparent group differences. The black students did not view their behavior as a cause for faculty disapproval, but rather took that disapproval as a racial slight (HEW Grant, 1975). White students viewed tutoring as a help (or at worst a minor inconvenience), and black students viewed it as a reflection upon their self-worth. The differences in class characteristics became a racial problem.

Personality Characteristics of the Faculty

Intelligence, motivation, and the latent identities of the faculty are important influences on the students' progress through the professional socialization stages.

It would be most desirable if all faculty members were extremely intelligent and motivated to make sure that all students received the best possible education, while including in their latent identity a commitment to a toleration of differences. Certainly not all faculty live up to this ideal; so in terms of structures conducive to professionalization, a variety of faculty again is an important component. Fortunately, not all faculty members resemble one another. Therefore, students who differ in age, race, ethnicity, and social class can still find role models. A student does not have to view every professor, instructor, or practitioner as an adequate role model; it is sufficient if only a few are not merely adequate but reliable and worthy of emulation.

Diversity in the faculty's latent identities (determining how they present themselves) increases the possibility that all students will find an appropriate role model. This faculty diversity will provide support for students through all the cognitive stages. Arrival at the cognitive Stage IV (interdependence) is facilitated by an appropriate role model who provides a road map to the desired goal. This role model is particularly important for those students who find the integration of professional and personal identities difficult.

SUMMARY

Structures that provide clearly defined paths from the beginning to the end of the professional educational process, suitable and varied role models for the students to emulate, an apprenticeship experience during which the students can test out their new skills under controlled circumstances, and cultural climates that are tolerant of individual differences, questioning, and testing, provide the desired structural supports and cultural conditions necessary for a good professional education.

Intelligence, motivation, and latent identities such as sex, age, race, and ethnicity also influence how students' progress through the stages to reach the goal of professional identification.

NOTES

1. By authoritarian climate we mean conditions in which students are expected to give unquestioning obedience to authority. The lack of authoritarianism does not imply excessive permissiveness or a lack of direction.

Part II

PROFESSIONAL SOCIALIZATION IN NURSING

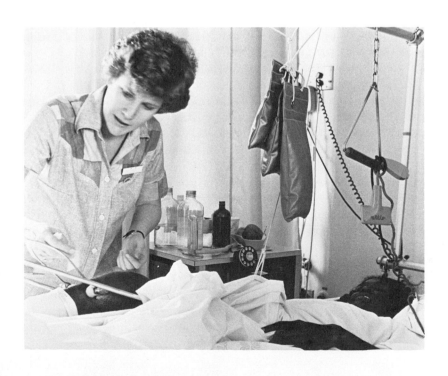

Chapter 4

HOW DO STUDENTS GROW?

An article by Corwin, Taves, and Haas (1961) indicates that there is great disillusionment with nursing as a career, and that nursing students are far more satisfied with nursing than are graduates. "High success as a nurse is significantly less satisfying than high success as a student nurse . . . Disillusionment with nursing is less consistently experienced by low success than high success personnel." (Success in this instance was measured by how students and graduate practitioners were rated by their clinical instructors and supervisors.) The authors attribute this to the fact that some characteristics such as professionalism and humanitarianism are stressed during education, while more tedious elements such as bureaucratic duties tend to be ignored. Other researchers have elaborated on this thesis (Kramer, 1974; Lewis, 1976; Fromm, 1977; Simms, 1977; Wang and Watson, 1977; Watson, 1977). Their studies indicate that the cause of disillusionment in nursing is rooted in the educational system and in problems in the socialization process.

In the previous chapters, a four stage model was presented to help analyze the professional socialization process students undergo in any professional education. The structural and cultural supports that enable students to progress through the stages were discussed, and nursing education was analyzed to see how nursing students might progress through these stages. Those chapters were theoretical and speculative; this chapter deals with the research that tells us about the reality of the educational process and discusses the specifics of the research into the cognitive, interactional, and personality spheres.

However, before attempting to analyze the socialization process in nursing, the confusion and controversy that surround the educational system must be analyzed. Montag (1951, 1964) attempted to clarify the situation and set forth the proposition that there are substantial differences between the technical and the professional aspects of nursing. Nursing functions are separated into three categories:

1. Simple or assisting functions, such as those performed by a nursing aide
2. Intermediate or technical functions, such as those performed by a "technical" nurse
3. Complex or professional functions performed by a university graduate "professional" nurse

The ANA (1965) formally accepted Montag's categories and proposed that all nursing education take place in colleges. The baccalaureate degree program would produce professional nurses, and junior colleges would award associate degrees to technical nurses. The role of the diploma program was virtually ignored, and the latent controversy in the educational system came to the surface.

The ANA Board of Directors, attempting to clarify and still some of the controversy aroused by the 1965 paper, in 1973 issued a statement that stressed the importance and value of service offered by graduates of diploma programs. The new statement, instead of stilling the controversy, intensified the confusion. Did this new paper indeed contradict the 1965 position paper? What was the diploma nurses' place? Would they be considered professional or technical?

The 1973 statement has been interpreted in various ways. Jacox (1976) asserts that it does not contradict the 1965 statement, but simply emphasizes a different aspect of professionalism. She feels the 1965 statement emphasizes upgrading the educational system; the 1973 statement emphasizes the necessary service aspect of the field. However, others view the 1973 statement as a step backwards. Armitage (1976) epitomizes this viewpoint: The paper is "a defensive reaction motivated by a well-intentioned desire to appease the sensitivities of a sector of the membership and to quiet unrest among diploma nursing students." At the 1978 ANA convention three resolutions were adopted. *Resolution 56: Identification and Titling of Establishment of Two Categories of Nursing Practice* proposes that the two categories be clearly identified and titled by 1980, and that the baccalaureate degree be the minimum preparation for entry into professional nursing by 1985. Two other statements, Resolution 57 and Resolution 58, call for a mechanism for establishing competency requirements for the two categories and increasing the accessibility of Career Mobility Programs in Nursing (programs that enable A.D. or diploma nurses to achieve the B.S.N.).

The split between the State Boards of Nursing Associations and the ANA (June 1976) hampers this progress. The state board associations must implement these resolutions via their state legislatures. Despite these obstacles and the resentment felt by diploma nurses forced back to school for the B.S.N. (Hillsmith, 1978), the B.S.N. will undoubtedly emerge as the minimum standard for the professional nurse. It is still unclear where this will leave today's diploma students and graduate nurses from diploma schools.

If the distinction between the technical and professional nurse had been implemented as neatly in reality as it is described in the 1965 ANA paper, ANA Resolutions 56 and 57 would have been unnecessary, and the three types of educational programs would have to be analyzed separately. Program length, curricula, and goals would be different, as would the student selection process and the process of professional socialization. However, there is continuing controversy over the practical reality of these distinctions.

Research on the attitudes of educators and employers and the selection process in nursing schools indicates that the three types of programs enroll, educate, and produce nurses who as groups are very much the same. Evidence is presented here to support our conclusion that the different programs are similar enough to be studied together.

Kohnke (1973) surveyed nursing educators to see how deans of A.D. and B.S.N. programs viewed their finished products. She asked the question, "Do nursing educators practice what is preached?" and found that they did not. The different programs had similar curricula and set similar goals for their graduates. Reichow and Scott (1976) surveyed employers, asking them to rate the effectiveness of graduates from the different programs, and found that employers viewed B.S.N., A.D., and diploma graduates as having similar skills and abilities. Beginning salaries were not based on type of degree (a good index that employers perceived few differences). Meleis and Farrel (1974) studied the attitudes of seniors from the three different types of programs to determine the quality of nursing care that could be expected from each type of graduate. Few differences between the seniors of the different types of programs were found. The intellectual potential and the responsibility toward patients did not vary. B.S.N. students showed only slightly higher leadership potential. These studies, despite the proposals in the ANA 1965 position paper and the alleged changes in nursing, show little change from earlier studies (Meyer, 1959; Dustan, 1964; Alutto, 1971; Ventura, 1976). The earlier studies had already indicated few differences in personality traits, intellectual qualities, professional attitudes, or the image of the nursing field held by the graduates of the different programs.

Kohnke (1973) states: "The curricular practice, as described by the majority of deans, is not, in fact, in line with that described in the literature." The curricula of A.D. and B.S.N. programs, Kohnke finds, are not clearly distinguished. Part of Kohnke's recommended solution is a transfer of emphasis in baccalaureate programs from technical skills to a broader knowledge base with an emphasis on planning and integrating concepts. The other part of the solution is limiting the roles of the A.D. nurse. Kohnke considers professional practice to be a mine field for A.D. nurses. Although they are trained to provide basic bedside care, they are frequently thrust into positions in which planning and conceptual skills are necessary to do the job competently. Their education has not prepared them for these positions. Sometimes they perform very well at great cost to themselves. Sometimes they are bewildered by the demands, and the resulting unsatisfactory performance is seen as a function of the inadequacy of the A.D. educational system, not the unrealistic job demands.

Studies of employer attitudes indicate that employers do not distinguish clearly between the roles of the B.S.N., the A.D., and the diploma nurse or between professional and technical functions. Indeed, Reichow and Scott (1976) found that the maxim "a nurse is a nurse is a nurse" holds true for employers. State Board exams are given to all three types of graduates and all become R.N.'s. Few of the employing institutions surveyed by Reichow and Scott made a dintinction between the type of preparation nurses receive. Nurses from different programs are given similar responsibilities and starting salaries. The majority of administrators from both large and small hospitals in the sample felt that, after a short time (between 6 months and 2 years) any differences in ability that may have existed at the beginning would disappear, and the two groups would be equal. Indeed, diploma nurses were preferred by administrators of small hospitals, even though there was a trend to regard baccalaureate nurses as showing more leadership. Reichow and Scott (1976) speculated that small hospitals prefer diploma nurses because they are thought to be more at ease in the hospital milieu than graduates of the other two programs. The selection process could conceivably differentiate the nursing programs from one another. If the B.S.N. schools recruited brighter and more assertive students than the A.D. or diploma programs, the socialization process in each program would proceed at different rates with different inherent problems. Meleis and Farrel (1974), addressing this question, tested senior nursing students and found:

> Students in the three types of programs . . . were essentially alike on intellectual characteristics, the consideration aspect of leadership and self-esteem. They were slightly above average, as compared with other college students in their concern for the feelings and welfare of people . . . and were inclined to be affiliate, trusting and ethical. They expressed similar degrees of consideration for subordinates and were inclined to respect their ideas. Baccalaureate students rated higher in the area of communication than associate degree or diploma seniors, and they were higher on the structure and autonomy factors of leadership. Diploma students placed highest value on research; baccalaureate students, lowest.*

From these studies we infer that it is possible to postulate a prototypical student nurse, Ms. Cherry Ames 1980, and examine the socialization process

---

*From Meleis, A.I., and Farrell, K.M. 1974. Operation concern: A study of senior nursing students in three nursing programs. *Nursing Research* 23:461-468.

in nursing as a whole. Differences between programs and differences that exist within the types of programs will be discussed in Chapter 5. This chapter is based on the assumption that Cherry Ames would encounter the same socialization process, if not curriculum, regardless of the type of school she attends. The process of this socialization will be examined by following the progress of a prototypical student through the four stages in the three spheres as presented in the socialization model in Chapter 2. In conclusion, this chapter examines how well prepared she will be upon graduation to assume her professional role and don the nursing mantle.

THE COGNITIVE SPHERE

How do aspiring nurses proceed through the cognitive stages? A survey of the literature and our research indicate that there are strong cultural and structural pressures to keep students in the first stage of dependency. First, let us examine the influence of nursing culture on the beginning student.

The tradition of obedience is immediately apparent. Group and Roberts (1974) call this "the ghost of the Crimea." The tradition of obedience in nursing is still alive and well. Jacox (1976) points out that although nursing has come a long way from the absolute militaristic obedience demanded in the 1890's, obedience is still seen as a virtue, especially for students. The media continues to portray nurses as physicians' handmaidens, and there are still jokes about the woman who enters nursing for the MRS. — M.D. degree. The culture sets the scene for the neophyte to enter Stage I very comfortable with the dependent role. Social stereotypes, the selection processes (both of the schools and of the individuals applying), and the expectations of the educators all combine to produce student comfort with dependence and corresponding problems for what is euphemistically labeled "an assertive student."

The neophyte nurse of the 1980s enters with a broader range of knowledge and is less constricted by her femaleness than those who preceded her. (Indeed, the changes in the student culture in the 1960s have made it difficult to find a truly obedient student.) However, in our study of diploma nurses, we found that 25% of the entering students in all eight schools were dependent, anxious students entering nursing to improve their self-concepts by becoming caretakers. They felt that becoming good nurses would enhance their ability to become good wives and mothers and allow them to put their religious beliefs into practice. This view of the field of nursing as enhancing their self-worth was highly correlated with the test (16 P.F.) profile of an anxious, neurotically dependent personality (see Appendix C for an explanation of the 16 P.F. test). This dependency and need also correlated positively with success in nursing education. The entire group that scored high on the 16 P.F. test graduated on schedule despite the 50% attrition rate in the class as a whole. This neurotic group comprised over 50% of the group that went into practice.

The success of the group with this set of attitudes should come as no surprise. Other researchers have found similar patterns and the core of the pattern is dependency, obedience, and low self-esteem. Nursing students often score high on the obedience scales of personality tests. Investigators in the 1960s (Reece, 1961; Katzell, 1968; Thurston and others, 1969) found that nursing students who were more tolerant of their own aggressions were more likely to become nonacademic dropouts. This same phenomenon was found in our study in a diploma school with a unique "open curriculum" that allowed students to proceed at their own pace. The curriculum encouraged autonomy, or Stage II, but the students who were more aware of and comfortable with their aggression were the most likely to leave.

In some schools, faculty members reinforce dependency by emphasizing the ultimate calamity—the death of a patient. This realistic professional problem becomes for entering students a nightmare that will expose their incompetence; for the faculty it becomes a club to enforce obedience. Information is presented with the warning, "If you don't learn this material right, someone may die." Olesen and Whittaker (1968) describe an instructor in a B.S.N. program who told a class that their math grades were too low for them to be allowed on the wards. The observer noted that the instructor was pleased when the students became visibly upset with this announcement. Obviously, instructors wish to prevent an "unsafe practitioner." Less obvious is the impact this has on the student or how it interferes with the student's desire to question material and act independently.

Unfortunately, the converse sometimes becomes the student's mode of thought. Students may think that if they memorize all the facts and learn by rote their patients will be safe. The fact that they will have to apply the facts at the proper time and use judgment does not occur to them. If it continues, this reliance on rote learning will be fatal to their becoming full-fledged professionals.

The structure of the educational system does little to break up the dependency encouraged by the nursing culture. Beginning basic science material is usually presented in large classes through routine lectures and by nonnursing faculty. The students are not shown the relationship between this required knowledge and their future activities as nurses. They learn by rote for grades that will allow them to continue in the program. There is a feeling of marking time—that courses merely serve as *rite de passage* and have no connection with nursing. The course material is perceived as irrelevant. This is especially true for diploma students who are anxious to skip theories and get to "the real stuff" (Mauksch, 1963).

An example of this attitude is illustrated by one group of students who seriously proposed that the reason for a much-hated 8:00 AM class was "to get them up early in the morning and assess whether they could stay alert in tedious surroundings." When they discussed this analysis with the administration, their motivations for studying nursing were questioned. The implication was that if the students were worthy of graduating, they would understand the reason for the course and not question its value.

Beginning medical students may also feel this way and learn only to pass exams (Becker and others, 1961). However, in medical school the student is not penalized for attitudes or feelings, and the irrelevance of the material serves as a spur for the student to go into the resistance of Stage II. In nursing, students are similarly resistant, but their resistance does not propel them into Stage II because the culture prevails against the structure. Nursing students feel that if they exhibit "too much" rebellion they will be "marked" when the time comes for clinical courses. They put up with marking time and try to look interested.

Another example of the repressive reactions provoked by negative/independence can be seen in the following incident: A student proved to her medical-surgical instructor that an open bar of soap could be a bacterial growth agent even if soap is a germicide. The student was not rewarded for good research or logical thought, although the instructor acknowledged she was right on her facts. Rather, when honors were presented to graduating seniors, she was passed over even though she had the highest grade point average. The reason was that her attitudes indicated to the faculty that she had problems with clinical skills; the "bar of soap" incident was cited to show she cared more for being right than contributing to class discussion. An incident such as this becomes part of the folklore of a school and cuts down cognitive resistance for years to come.

Therefore, the negative/independence stage is—if not completely suppressed—at least not allowed active expression. This does not provide a good foundation for the next stage.

The structures of nursing programs provide a good basis for Stage III (mutuality), where divergent thought processes are experienced and the selection of alternatives must be made. Nursing's apprentice education allows them to practice the behavior they will utilize as professionals. In their clinical experience, students do apply in "real" situations the knowledge they have learned. They receive their clinical experience in small groups and build from the simple activities to the more complex skills. Students can and do study together, forming groups that permit cognitive feedback and protect their self-esteem against instructor criticism.

The curricula and educational goals are oriented toward producing individuals who can make good professional judgments, think abstractly, and apply concretely. Unfortunately, the programmatic structure cannot prevail against the nursing culture. No matter how well the philosophy of education is defined or how well integrated the curricula are, education will be transmitted through the culture bearers. Faculty still tend to assume that there are right answers for every question, and students are expected to respond with correct data stated in a "proper" way. This atmosphere overrides the structural props, leaving the students with the same cognitive attitudes they had in Stage I (although they now have an expanded data base). The students may try to provide a solid front in seminars and clinical conferences and justify rebellion against the faculty standards. This is usually short-lived because the faculty again holds the ultimate trump card. All they have to do is to remind the students of the possibility of a patient's death, and they will inhibit the students' progress to any stage past dependence. It is not that nursing students do not try to progress to Stages II and III or that the supportive structures are not there. Rather, the culture bearers (that is, the educators and role models) prevent such progress.

Stage IV in the cognitive sphere is interdependence. It may be expected, according to a philosophy of education, that this stage will be reached upon graduation. Employers, however, expect that it will be some time after graduation before the new graduate is comfortable in his or her role. The progression to role comfort (if indeed it is ever acquired) depends on idiosyncratic variables in the first job placement. Since the nursing field is in conflict about the amount of autonomy and initiative that should be permitted a graduate nurse, new graduates cannot expect structural supports for their struggles.

Nursing educators and administrators realize that autonomy is a problem for nursing. Much of the nursing literature examines the problem of autonomy. Many believe that the nurse-practitioner will solve this problem. The new status of the nurse in the 1980s as proposed by the ANA (see Chapters 5 and 10) may encourage the new gradutes to be in Stage IV. However, if they are products of an educational system that inhibits the negative/independence of Stage II and the mutuality of Stage III, Stage IV interdependence will be impossible to reach.

INTERACTIONAL SPHERE

How do students learn to behave in a manner appropriate to their profession and emulate those already in the field? In the interactional sphere, as well as in the cognitive, there are cultural norms that interfere with the students' progress through the stages.

The first cultural barrier is society's view of the nursing profession. It is apparent to students that society does not respect the technical knowledge base of the nurse the way it does that of the physician. This is obvious in the media stereotypes, which are reinforced in nursing texts. Nursing texts are likely to have a primerlike appearance, with "cute" pictures and captions, in sharp contrast to the more technical and scholarly medical texts that will be used for reference. Some universities and junior colleges have basic science courses designed specifically for nurses that are not acceptable for regular college credit. This signals the students that nursing students are considered incapable of understanding the regular college level courses. Some students may appreciate the fact that nursing is "easier," but the brighter and more assertive students tend to feel denigrated.

Another cultural barrier that supports dependency and hinders progress through the other stages is the perceived authoritarian atmosphere of the faculty and administration. Many schools and administrations are aware of the problems caused by authoritarian education, and much is written in nursing literature on ways to combat this influence. Some schools are turning to the "open curriculum," in which students set the pace of the learning; many schools try to involve students at the various levels of decision-making in both academic and social matters. Certainly all schools try to provide protected learning experiences for the neophyte and assure that the first assigned cases do not overtax the students' skills and cause unnecessary trauma. However, the nursing culture cannot be denied. With all the concern about pressuring students and encouraging autonomy, there is still the tacit assumption that there is one right way to do things—any other is a mistake, and mistakes kill! Faculty and administration cannot free the students from this spectre because they are bound by it themselves. Competent graduates in the field are frequently at the mercy of this idea and strive to become error-free caretakers who can do anything—in other words, "supernurses."

Cohen and Orlinsky (1977) discuss this problem extensively in their paper on work stress in critical care units. They found that nurses tend to become physically ill rather than admit that they are weak or need help. When veteran nurses are convinced that they must do everything perfectly or the patient will die, the student feels compelled to do likewise. Long before a fastfood chain of restaurants used it, the advertising campaign that nursing had taken as its professional stance was "We do it all for you." This ideology implicit in the professional culture is transmitted to the students. Interestingly, Olesen and Whittaker (1968) suggest that the punitive aspects of this ideology are mitigated in the B.S.N. university-based programs. However, the explicit examples they choose to illustrate this point do not suggest mitigation, they suggest authoritarianism. This emphasis on perfection pressures students to stay in Stage I and avoid any show of autonomy.

In the interactional sphere, structural aspects also reinforce the dependency of Stage I. Entering students are primarily high school graduates who probably have had some medical-based work experiences. The students who have worked in a hospital setting appear to adopt the professional nursing values more easily, but the experience is not an adequate preparation for initiation into the nursing role. Compared to other aspiring professionals, nurses have relatively little anticipatory socialization. (Anticipatory socialization is the process of anticipating a future role, thinking about its facets, and beginning to enact the behavior and adopt the values of the future profession.) This lack appears odd since the literature indicates that many students select nursing at an early age and report that they have always wanted to be nurses. However, in nursing, anticipatory socialization does not provide adequate preparation because the image of nursing to which they aspire is a childish one inferred from stereotypes and the media. Nothing is required of students before actual entrance into the educational program. Medical and law students may be similarly influenced by cultural stereotypes in their occupational choice, but they have 3 or 4 years of preparation before qualifying for entrance into law or medical schools. During this time, they have a chance to investigate the question, "Is the profession worth this?" If the answer is "yes," they can then begin anticipating the proper role behaviors. By the time aspiring nurses can ask the same question, they are in the midst of the professional education where proper role behavior is demanded, not developed. They have not developed internal guidelines to help them function, so they must rely on the guidelines supplied by others.

Another structural support for dependence is supervised dormitory living. Although the trend in recent years is away from *in loco parentis* dormitory living, it still exists, particularly in hospital-based schools. In such situations, dependency may be extreme. The close quarters allow the faculty access to the students' private nonclassroom behavior. They can control the hours students keep and their dress and personal appearance—aspects usually ignored in other educational institutions. This situation resembles in part the process of induction into the military, where every aspect of the person's life comes under scrutiny (Zurcher, 1967). Dependency is extended to all aspects of the "boot's" life, as those in authority attempt to restructure the civilian personality into one that is a "military" personality. As recently as 1969, nursing enforced dependency in similar ways with rules against student marriages, long hair, unkempt appearance, and other behavior not considered ladylike or worthy of the "Nightingale ideal." Even today many educators bemoan the passing of those times when everything that happened during the educational time span was considered a nursing experience and subject to faculty review. Since dormitory living is now most prevalent in diploma schools with their hospital base, it is in this type of program that the cultural supports for dependency remain the strongest. The different types of educational programs do not differ much in their cultural expectations which produce dependency, but it is the diploma schools that provide the most structural support for this first stage.

To move to the second stage of resistance and become rebellious in such an atmosphere is to play with fire. College and graduate students can "hassle" instructors and only risk their final grades. Even this risk is minimized if there are departmental examinations or alternative sections of the course. The nursing student is told, occasionally explicitly, that her attempts to question, clarify, or disagree with the instructors make her clinically unsafe. Even if the student is unusually good academically, a rebellious attitude may cause the faculty to judge her clinically unsafe and unable to function with patients. To rebel is to risk too much.

In the 1940s, Cherry Ames did not have the problem of dealing with her rebelliousness in an authoritarian atmosphere. She was not rebellious, and the faculty and administration understood that. Her problems arose when her dedication and obedience to the system were misunderstood. The misunderstanding could be cleared up by explanation — there were no deep-seated motivational problems to be solved.

Nursing is moving away from demands for obedience (Jacox, 1976), and this shows up first in the selection process. This movement in selection was forced by the youth of today — the truly obedient are harder to find. However, since the faculty members are products of their education (which took place before these changes), the educational process still bears strong similarities to the system encountered by Cherry Ames. Modern students struggle with the culture of a different era and outmoded structures.

In spite of all these cultural and structural factors encouraging dependence, there are elements engendered by the same system that encourage resistance. One is student discomfort with the role models, which stems from two sources. The first source is the very authoritarianism that fosters the dependence and compliance of the first stage. Authoritarianism and perfectionism are inevitably resented, and it is difficult to remain compliant and dependent if the authoritarianism of one's mentors is resented. The second is the difficulty in finding models who present appropriate and varied presentations of the role. Nursing students (like medical students) see teachers who probably are not practitioners. This leaves the students feeling alienated from the field at the beginning of the educational process. When students begin their apprenticeship, these problems with finding appropriate role models may intensify rather than decrease because of the discrepancy between the academic educator and the practitioner. Students find identifying with the academic individual (who, after all, holds the power) easier, but then they must close their eyes to the practice on the units. Exposure to this discrepancy does give the student the view that alternative courses of action are possible, but the instructors' insistence that ward personnel are not acting properly frequently does away with this advantage. The implication is that if the students are going to become good professionals, they will ignore what they see — or, if necessary, inveigh against it when they graduate. However, the result of these contradicting influences may mean a lack of identification with either role model and a corresponding boost into Stage II and resistance.

The other structural support for resistance comes from a two-edged sword — dormitory living. Dormitory living fosters dependency via faculty control over nonacademic facets of student life, but students who live in close contact can easily form a student culture that can be used to resist the official culture. Gripe sessions, study sessions, and social events, allow opportunities for student interaction outside the classroom. The students may use these as vehicles to solidify their discontents and gain group support for resistance. There is strength and safety in numbers. "After all," the students rationalize, "they can't throw out a whole class."

However, overt rebellions occur only under extreme conditions, such as open expressions of racism by a white faculty to a primarily black class. Usually the demonstration of resistance is more subtle. In *The Silent Dialogue* (1968), Olesen and Whittaker discuss how students in the B.S.N. program learn to give the expected answers and present approved attitudes to the faculty, while keeping their thoughts and ideas to themselves. Olesen and Whittaker dislike the idea of students being "con men" (we trust that today, with a raised consciousness, they would say "con artists"), but acknowledge that this may be part of the educational process. In this conning of the faculty and presenting what is necessary to pass, nursing students resemble medical students who study to pass a test. The difference is that the nursing students' attitudes, as well as their knowledge and performance, are under scrutiny, and they are forced to comply at all levels. The Cherry Ames of the 1980s marches into a system still autocratic at the core and cannot indulge in even covert resistance for any length of time. The structures and cultural supports that foster movement into Stage II are almost completely stifled by lack of opportunity for expression and the strong sanctions against questioning and assertiveness.

How do students cope with Stage III when Stage II has been so difficult? In Stage III (mutuality) the students should gather in groups, try on the professional role and receive feedback on their behaviors and attitudes from their peers and superiors. All types of nursing education programs include an apprenticeship experience, although it is longest in the diploma programs. The students are expected to do what nurses do, but they do not have legal responsibility for their actions. Their duties progress from the simple to the complex, and professional behavior is demanded of them. The students have a chance to interact with physicians and patients, trying out attitudes and ways of behaving that they can incorporate into their professional identity. They can evaluate their role models by getting together and talking about their instructors and the graduate nurses on their units. In short, this stage should occur naturally since the proper structural components exist for its realization.

However, students are expected to play Stage III with Stage I demeanor — subservience. The cultural support for Stage III is lacking even if the structural supports are all in place. The discrepancy between clinical and classroom instructors, which may have pushed the students into covert resistance, interferes with Stage III. It is difficult for students to identify with the practitioners if they are told that the practitioners are professionally inadequate. The idealism of classroom instructors leads them to denigrate their practitioner peers, and this leaves students confused. It is difficult to identify with unacceptable role models, but less than useful to identify with the academic role models if one is to become a practitioner. What will be the reference group necessary to Stage III? Peers are not enough; students should feel that those already in the role are becoming acceptable. In this situation, establishing a reference group is difficult.

At Stage III, students who have gone through the resistance stage under-cover now emerge as leaders. These leaders do experience anticipatory socialization by trying on the role of graduate nurse. They enjoy this and their own expanded knowledge base so much that they frequently view faculty and practitioners alike as "dim bulbs." They will become the right type of nurse — professional and comfortable in their roles. In this they are reminiscent of Handlin's (1952) description of the children of immigrants who became their own cultural forebears to fit into the new dominant culture. Many senior nursing students do this for themselves and foresee their graduate identity as different from the instructors and practitioners they have encountered during their educational experience. Unfortunately, becoming one's own role model promotes a great deal of inner anxiety. Erikson (1950) describes these individuals as always unsure of their acceptance by their neighbors. Many students, while certain they are behaving more professionally than their educators, are nevertheless unsure of their acceptance by colleagues and clients.

Sometimes the staff will have one "young rebel" with whom the students can identify and expound on their theories of what nursing should be and relate the problems of living up to their ideals. The students often emulate this staff member. When this happens, Stage III is assured. Unfortunately, having this type of staff member around is "the luck of the draw." It is not institutionalized or guaranteed.

Theoretically, Stage IV (interdependence) is attained upon graduation, but in practice all agree that professional practice must take place first. It is 6 months to licensure and perhaps longer for orientation after the first job placement. New graduates are protected and watched with apprehension. Because of the problems in Stages II and III, resolution of Stage IV becomes idiosyncratic. Some students pull themselves through the stages; some programs have supports that help pull students through. Some students progress to Stage IV quickly once in the work role; others drop out in frustration. Unfortunately, it is left to chance whether the first job placement will have the conditions necessary for fostering this final transition.

THE PERSONALITY SPHERE

What affect does the socialization process have on the self-concept and personality of the nursing student? Erikson (1950) hypothesizes that identification with an occupational role or profession "ties up the loose ends" of the individual's identity and helps integrate all stages of development and concepts of self that have preceded this stage. This work identity propels the adolescent into adulthood. Does assuming the identity of a professional nurse do this for the newly graduated student? Does she feel confidence in herself as a professional and does this identification with the professional role help her in the transition from adolescence to adulthood? Corwin, Taves, and Haas (1961), Kramer (1974), and others indicate that although students may enter nursing expecting this to happen (one-fourth of our sample of 800 nurses did), few graduates think that becoming a professional nurse helps them formulate an adult identity.

Why is this so? Nursing has come a long way from the time when schools advertised for plain women who wished to serve. The nursing student today will probably be offered a variety of role models with whom to identify. Nursing curricula are constantly being revised to offer students more autonomy and initiative in their educational experiences. However, there is still professional disillusionment on the part of graduates and a great deal of literature calling for more autonomy and initiative in the nursing role.

Perhaps the answer to the problems in the personality sphere resides in the fact that the "ghost of the Crimea" has not been exorcised. Group and Roberts (1974) coined this phrase and are particularly concerned with the authoritarianism in nursing education. They state:

> Few people would dispute the fact that an authoritarian structure is not conducive to a positive educational experience. But unfortunately, when nursing education shifted its professional learning base from service to educational institutions, it maintained the authority model derived from the hospital bureaucracy and from military organizations. This situation was reinforced by the fact that American universities and colleges themselves were for a long time based on Prussian models of education which were primarily authoritarian in structure and operation.
>
> Nurses were thus caught within, or between, two male-dominated, authoritarian institutions, and the restricting and constricting influence of this situation continues. In a hospital, dedicated to the sustenance of life, this situation is disastrous; in education, dedicated to the free exploration of ideas, it is intolerable.*

To the young student, expecting to acquire the professional role, it is both confusing and dismaying. Frequently, students feel called upon to identify with what the faculty perceives to be "an ideal nurse," ignoring students' individual identities. Here interactional problems impinge on the personality development. Werner (1973) sees a credibility gap between what educators profess and what they practice, and suggests that this leads students to brand faculty as hypocrites. Werner reminds faculty that they must show students

*From Group, T.M., and Roberts, J.I. 1974. Exorcising the ghosts of the Crimea. *Nursing Outlook* 22(6):369.

how to integrate the female and professional nursing roles by giving them opportunities to work through the problem, not just telling them about it:

> Our students watch us very closely, not only in the classroom or clinical setting, but in the halls, in the coffee shop and cafeteria, in meetings, at student-faculty affairs. Students know a great deal about us and whether or not we are comfortable with this, there is little we can do about it, other than to keep reminding ourselves that anything a student learns about us—it may be good, it may be bad—stands a chance of being incorporated into that student's value system.
>
> This, as I see it, is the challenge for faculty in professional socialization. Programs, curricula and clinical experience are obviously important, but the individual teacher is the critical element.*

The faculty does indeed play a crucial role in the professionalization process, but how does one model an identity with which one is not yet comfortable? Group and Roberts (1974) point out that nursing faculty tend to be isolated from universities' power structures, as are nursing administrators in hospital settings. Grandjean, Aiken, and Bonjean (1976) find that nursing educators rate teaching, supportive colleagues, keeping their clinical knowledge current, and faculty autonomy as the most important aspects of their jobs. Williamson (1972) and Batey (1969) have addressed at length the problem of the nursing faculty within a university system. Both emphasize that the faculty member is caught between two normative systems: the service-oriented, bureaucratic hospital and the professional, autonomous university. Batey states:

> The entrance of various service-oriented fields into the university has contributed to an incongruity between the university's goals and those of the new participants. With specific reference to nursing faculty, I attribute this situation to three factors: (1) while current patterns of undergraduate nursing education emphasize the creative acts of patient services, they provide little or no formal socialization to the norms associated with discovery and transmission of new knowledge; (2) the nurse faculty member has acquired through formal and informal processes their views and values and (3) current patterns of graduate education in nursing provide insufficient opportunities for acquisition of values and behaviors associated with the discovery and transmission of new knowledge.**

The result, according to Batey, is:

> Many nursing faculty members continue to operate according to the norms of behavior familiar from another position in another type of organization—that of a nurse in a hospital . . . They continue to expect remunerative and promotional rewards more for conscientious fulfillment of assigned responsibilities

---

*From M. Werner, 1973. Professional socialization of nurses: A faculty member's view. *Journal of the New York State Nurses Association* 4(4):25.
**From Batey, M.V. 1969. The two normative worlds of the university nursing faculty. *Nursing Forum* 5(1):15.

of teaching and administrative duties than for discovery and transmission of new knowledge.*

Williamson (1972), in "The Conflict-Producing Role of the Professionally Socialized Nurse-Faculty Member," shows how this problem alienates young faculty members and, consequently, students:

> Many "old school" nursing leaders holding responsible administrative positions in the university setting find it difficult to accept the motivations of the professionally socialized faculty member who is breaking out of the traditional mold. In turn, the faculty member is finding it equally difficult to pursue a professional career within the confines of an environment alien to her expectations . . . Faculty is responsible for socializing the student to the professional value system but to be able to socialize, one must be socialized to the set of norms considered acceptable to that role.**

As a result, the administrations of nursing departments do not resemble the administrations in other departments, and nursing administrators frequently concentrate on keeping their own house in order without learning the administrative skills needed to survive in the university setting (such as how to become members of committees determining budget, tenure, positions, etc.). Williamson also points out that nursing administrators and sometimes nursing faculty tend toward a mother-surrogate role rather than toward the consultant and coordinator role used by other disciplines. Nursing students who receive their first 2 years of education within the total university environment find the mother-surrogate role presented by nursing faculty to be a surprise and sometimes an unpleasant shock. Indeed, Williamson considers much of the internal conflict in all nursing organizations to be a result of the differences in these two orientations:

> As long as this diversity and conflict (that is, mother-surrogate versus consultant) occur, we can assume two possible consequences: (1) nursing will not be totally accepted as an integral part of professional education, and (2) nursing students will remain confused in their roles as professionals and severely limited in carrying out in practice the tenets of professionalism.†

The problems between the authoritarianism of the old-line nursing educator and university norms are illustrated by this example: A nursing department brought in a new Ph.D. to resolve this conflict between university and nursing administrators. The Dean of Graduate Studies had demanded from the head of the nursing department a revised curriculum and apprenticeship experience that would reflect the university philosophy of research and

---

*From Batey, M.V. 1969. The two normative worlds of the university nursing faculty. *Nursing Forum* 5(1):15.
**From Williamson, J.A. 1972. The conflict-producing role of the professionally socialized nurse-faculty member. *Nursing Forum* 11(4):357.
†From Williamson, J.A. 1972. *Nursing Forum* 11(4):366.

promote autonomy and initiative in clinical situations. The new Ph.D. in nursing designed a curriculum more conceptual and less concrete in nature and found a series of clinical placements that would provide experiences where students could exercise autonomy and initiative. The Dean of Graduate Studies was pleased with the changes and commended the Ph.D. However, the new Ph.D. was horrified when she found that no arrangements had been made to implement either the new curriculum or the new placements. The nursing chairperson viewed the revisions as interesting but impractical. The staff would not be able to supervise the students adequately in the proposed system, and the students might make clinical errors. If they did, patients would die. The new professional was now a "young rebel" and protested the action vigorously in the faculty forum. Her contract was not renewed at the end of the year. As the department chairperson phrased it, "You are an excellent academic nurse, but I doubt that you really understand the problems of clinical safety, and this could be dangerous for the students. Besides, your peers are afraid of you because you always question their knowledge."

It is not only the students who are at the mercy of the authoritarian culture or the "ghost of the Crimea." Faculty members frequently feel that they do not have the autonomy necessary to do their jobs well. How can they then model an autonomous professional identity for students? Williamson's point is well taken. Nursing students are frequently confused as they try to advance through Stage II of resistance to Stage III of mutuality and group support, where they can try on for size the professional nursing image. Their confusion mirrors that of the young faculty member who experiences the same problems.

CONCLUSION

There is little point in speculating on what happens to the personality in Stages III and IV, when so much evidence exists that Stage II presents an insurmountable problem for students and faculty alike. In reviewing my data on the 800 diploma nurses and the literature on personality characteristics of nursing students, it becomes apparent that nursing students have problems with autonomy and are more passive than other college students. The literature on nursing educators, stemming mostly from high status B.S.N. schools, indicates that faculty and administrators in nursing have trouble with their own autonomy within the health care system. The faculty could not provide a safe climate for Cherry Ames in the 1970s to trust and work out her resistance, progressing through the stages of autonomy and initiative, because they had problems of their own in these areas. The bright, inquisitive, and challenging student who exhibits Stage II resistance with a flourish is a threat to the careful cover placed over the dissonance between what faculty wish for themselves and what they perceive themselves as receiving.

However, this is not inevitable. Some very capable nurses manage to become autonomous and powerful in the complex arenas of university and hospital politics. However, they do this on the basis of idiosyncratic skills and personality variables; there is no prototypical way to gain power, and such powerful women are often considered "one of a kind." Some become powerful through skill at the "doctor-nurse game" (Stein, 1971), in which they can impart information to physicians and administrators without appearing to violate the tradition of subservience in the female or nursing role. If they become good enough at this game, soon many decisions will be delegated and finally the good player ends up with most of her unit, however large and complex, under her control. Others become "Grand Dames," an approach that is more successful after middle age. Nurses cannot, while still in their twenties, look down their noses at the physician, provost or president and say, "Young man, where did you ever get that idea?" An example of this approach was given by one nursing administrator who, when informed by the hotel manager that all convention-rate rooms were taken and that she and her staff would have to pay full rates, looked at the bill and then asked, "Young man, do you think we were planning to acquire the property?" Scaled-down rates were quickly obtained. Said the 19-year-old student representative, "Gee, I wish I could do that." At her age she could not. Interestingly, many of the most forceful members of the nursing profession recall their younger years as difficult — not only for them but for their faculty and educational institutions as well.

Unfortunately, these nursing administrators who have managed to become autonomous and reach Stage IV of interdependence are of little use as role models to the students aspiring to the professional role. If the students perceive the nursing faculty as stepchildren within the hospital or university milieu, they cannot trust their role models. What safety can the impotent provide? If the nurse has acquired power through adroit use of the doctor-nurse game, students fear her as a model. The game based on manipulation precludes trusting the individuals involved. Someone who can manipulate physicians can also manipulate students. The Grand Dame stance may invoke admiration but only when the attitude is focused on others. The implicit authoritarianism in this approach makes it potentially dangerous for the student. The student may be more admiring than fearful, but identification is precluded by an approach so obviously age-related. The implication is that while some students may indeed reach Stage IV in all three spheres, this is a rarity, resulting from the personality of the student and not encouraged by the cultural climate.

What happens upon graduation? How does the newly graduated student adjust to her chosen profession? To the dismay of many, she may not adjust. She may leave the field within the year (Kramer, 1974). The new graduate is technically competent, since dependency does not interfere with acquisition of the knowledge base.

However, the student's reaction to the first job does interfere with the socialization process. Kramer (1974) reports that newly graduated nurses experience "reality shock," demonstrated by the students' dismay upon finding so many bureaucratic duties. Corwin (1961) had previously reported the same phenomenon, calling it professional disillusionment. Observation of numerous students from a variety of programs entering the work role had led me to suspect that "reality shock" is not the result of a sudden confrontation with an unknown, the bureaucratic system. (After all, even in a university setting, nursing is an apprentice profession. How can a new graduate, after spending at least 2 years on various units in a hospital, not know about the hospital as a system and the authoritarianism associated with the bureaucracy of the health care delivery?) Perhaps the shock results from meeting a reality only too well known. Students tend to believe that if they can stick it out to graduation, it will be "all right"—in other words, they will be in control of themselves. Without having to answer to an authoritarian system, they can go through their questioning stage without being frightened.

The shock comes when they find that the total system reflects the same problems inherent in their education. The health care system demands that they produce as professionals and take responsibility for their judgments while maintaining subservient attitudes. Some leave because this demand is too great. Others say it is only a job and do what they can to get by, ignoring the "calling" aspects of the profession and making themselves objects of scorn to their peers.

As one recent dropout (preparing for a legal career) put it:

> Nursing, who needs it? If you do a really good job that satisfies you, the administration is on your back for devoting too much time to one patient and not filling in piddling little forms. Your peers are mad because you show them up. Most just want to sit on their asses and view you as a rate breaker. The doctors make snide remarks like, "You are too pretty to be a ball-buster,"—meaning, "don't question me." How can I take good care of his patient if I don't ask questions, and why does he think it's his patient? I spend more time with the patient and will be the one there if something goes wrong. The great M.D. will probably be on the golf course. Patients always arrest on Wednesday and every (expletive deleted) M.D. in this place is on the fairway then.

Nursing position papers call for recognizing the value of the questioning and assertive student and demand more autonomy for the practitioner. Well they might, for with this former nursing student, the legal profession's gain is the nursing profession's loss. The student graduated first in her class and is now repeating this performance in law school. Her hospital performance was outstanding. She reorganized many procedures on her unit, which resulted in the administration's deploring her unorthodoxy even though the life expectancy of patients increased. Profane and difficult, she was early spotted as a problem and sent for counseling, which enabled her to survive the student system. Later, she underwent therapy and left nursing.

At present the enforced dependency initiated by the educational program and perpetuated by the health care system cannot produce and retain self-confident professionals who feel accepted by their clients, peers, and other health care professionals. Although nursing education has made every effort to structure Stage III into the program, problems in Stage I and Stage II prevent real mutuality, and without that there can be no true professional identity. Since students are denied rebellion, they fail to become autonomous, and the industry of Stage III reflects compliance rather than autonomy and initiative. Students who learn a professional role using Stage I demeanor emerge looking and acting like robots, unable to deal with new situations. They are not attached to their professional roles because the period of autonomy that is crucial for the integration of the self and the professional role is missing. The dropout rate of licensed nurses attests to this aspect of the problem. If students flee from reality shock and role conflict in the professional field, the socialization process has not properly run its course. Much must be done if nursing students are to become truly professional.

NOTES

1. This last finding is of particular interest since one prime argument for university-based programs is that these programs inculcate a research orientation. This study casts doubt on this assumption.

Chapter 5

COMPARISON OF NURSING EDUCATION PROGRAMS

In Chapter 4 the socialization process in nursing education as a whole was analyzed without differentiating its impact on the different kinds of nursing programs. It was decided that this type of analysis was justified after reviewing the literature on the differences between graduates of respective programs. Researchers find a blurring of distinction between programs (Reichow and Scott, 1976; Kohnke, 1973). Neither the deans of different types of programs nor the hospital directors who hire nurses think graduates of the respective programs are substantially different. From these and other studies, we deduced that the socialization process is similar in all programs because of the all-pervasive nursing culture, and that it is not significantly modified by the particular educational structure.

Although the various programs produce similar graduates, the programs are far from identical. Since a different amount of time is required to complete the programs (2 years for the A.D. program, 3 years for the diploma program, and 4 years for the B.S.N.), and there are differences in staffs' philosophy and curricula, it is not surprising to learn that investigators report differences in cognitive ability, socioeconomic status, age, attitudinal traits, and personality traits among students enrolled in the three types of programs. These differences will affect the process of socialization, although not necessarily the final product.

This chapter reviews the relevant literature on intellectual, demographic, and personality variables of nursing students in the three types of nursing programs and then relates these variables to the different spheres in the socialization process (cognitive, interactional, and psychological) to assess how the differences, if any, will affect the professional socialization process in each type of educational program. Finally, the literature will be examined for evidence of Stage II, resistance, in nursing education.

WHO GOES INTO EACH TYPE OF PROGRAM?

The greatest difference found among programs is in the type of student recruited into each program. Students vary along intellectual, demographic, attitudinal, and personality variables. Before reporting the extensive literature on this topic there is a necessary caveat: Most studies are of seniors who would undoubtedly reflect both the selection and the socialization process. It is important to begin, therefore, with the studies that report the differences among entering students.

In 1971 Wren did an extensive analyses of freshman students in all three types of programs in the state of Georgia. The study included 19 different variables, including demography, aptitude, and motivation for those entering nursing. Three prototypes were drawn up to describe the typical female nursing student in each program. These prototypes are as follows:

1. Baccalaureate student: This student is unmarried; willing to travel some distance from home to attend a university school of nursing; is financing her education from personal and family funds or from part time work while in nursing school; has parents who are high school graduates and possibly college gradutes; ranked in the upper fourth of her high school graduating class; has an SAT score of 972; gave some thought to continuing education after graduation; was influenced in her career choice by a high school counselor or a nurse; has previous work experience, possibly in some type of nursing function; chooses nursing as a career because of a desire to help people and for personal advancement; and chooses her nursing school because of its reputation and curriculum.

2. Diploma student: This student entered nursing immediately after high school; is not married; is willing to attend a hospital school of nursing some distance from her hometown; receives financial support from personal and family funds; has parents who are high school graduates, college graduates, or have some college education; ranked in the upper 50% of her high school class; has an SAT score of 899; plans to continue her education after graduation; was most influenced in her choice of nursing by a nurse; has had no previous college work before entering nursing school; has worked part time before entering nursing school, probably as a nurse aide; chooses nursing as a career because of a desire to help people or for personal advancement; and

chooses her present school because of the educational experience it
provided.

3. Associate Degree student: This student is older than the other types of
    students; is married or was once married; finances her education from
    personal funds, family funds, or part time work while in school; has
    parents who did not finish high school; probably ranked in the upper
    half of her high school class but might have ranked in lower half; has
    an SAT score of 822; is more likely to plan on working in a hospital
    after graduation than are graduates of the other two programs; is
    thinking of continuing her education after graduation; was recruited
    into nursing by a nurse or a nursing school recruiter; did not have
    college work before entering nursing school but might have been an
    L.P.N.; chooses nursing as a career to help people and because she
    has always wanted to be a nurse; and chooses her present school
    because of its low cost and proximity to home.*

These differences in socioeconomic status, age, and age-related variables
such as family and children have been confirmed by other researchers (Dustan,
1964; Stromberg, 1976). Bayer and Schoenfeldt (1970) drew a sample of over
1000 students from nursing programs throughout the nation to counteract the
regional bias that might account for Wren's findings. In this study, social class
was the single strongest and differentiating variable between B.S.N. and
diploma students. The diploma students came from lower social-status homes
than did the B.S.N. students.

Wren (1971) found significant differences in aptitude as reflected by SAT
scores. Baccalaureate students' scores were about 150 points higher than the
A.D. students' scores, and diploma students' scores were midway between the
two groups. Dustan (1964) also found differences between programs;
however, the direction of the difference is different. In Dustan's sample, A.D.
students' scores on aptitude tests were the highest, and diploma students' the
lowest. Dustan also found differences in intellectual interest patterns. A.D.
students exhibited the most scientific and intellectual interests and diploma
students demonstrated the lowest. In contrast to these two studies, Bayer and
Schonfeldt (1970) found negligible differences between B.S.N. and diploma
students in five out of six aptitude and achievement tests.

Why are there such discrepancies? Perhaps it is because each researcher
has a piece of the total picture and mistakes this for the whole configuration,
similar to the blind men examining the elephant.

Dustan (1964) found the age difference between the A.D. and the
diploma nurse to be highly significant. The effect of this age difference could
account for the differences in aptitude and intellectual interest. Aptitude and

*Modified from Wren, G. 1971. Some characteristics of freshman students in baccalaureate,
diploma and associated degree nursing programs. *Nursing Research* 17:140-145.

vocabulary could have increased with age and experience. Indeed, in this sample, unlike Wren's, A.D. students had more education than the other groups. Wren's sample, drawn from schools in Georgia, might reflect the state of nursing education in Georgia rather than in the nation. Bayer and Schoenfeldt had a nationwide sample, but they compared only B.S.N. and diploma graduates. Differences in research focus and sampling techniques might also account for the differences cited in those studies.

Another problem not dealt with by any of these researchers is the immense variation between schools within these type of programs. This is especially true of diploma programs. Alutto and others (1971) found in testing for personality characteristics that diploma students show tremendous variation, individually and among schools. My data from nine different classes in seven schools show that schools, and even different classes in one school, vary tremendously as to demographic factors, intellectual variables, and personality characteristics. Jones (1976) also found that class level and demographic factors influenced his findings, which indicated that B.S.N. students scored higher on aptitude tests. When these factors were controlled, the differences between students in the various programs were not as significant.

The difficulties and uncertainties of research on the usual academic aptitude predictors are compounded when researchers try to include measures of creativity in assessing the differences among the various programs. Creativity is defined in these studies as an aspect of intellect (Guildford, 1967). It is a thought process in which there is an ability to give alternative answers rather than converging on one right answer or procedure. There is not much research in this area, since creativity is not necessarily related to a successful practice.

One of the few studies on creativity in nursing did find significant differences on several measures of creativity (Ventura and Meyers, 1976). However, the fact that students from each type of program scored highest on one of the measured components casts doubt on the validity of the findings, since the measures are usually used only as contributors to a total score. The originality scale that deals most definitively with Guildford's concept of convergence shows no differences among groups.

The existing research into differences between students in the three types of programs does not reveal the precise nature of the group differences. It is not clear whether the *inter*group differences in each program are such that *intra*group differences cannot be assessed. The diploma schools I studied varied so much from one another on academic, demographic, and personality variables that it would be difficult to compare these diploma programs with the baccalaureate programs in the same geographic area. The differences among the diploma schools would undoubtedly outweigh whatever differences could be found between the diploma programs and baccalaureate programs. Despite this difficulty, this section assesses the spheres of socialization to see which, if any, differences can be found that will affect the socialization process in each type of educational program.

THE SOCIALIZATION PROCESS
IN NURSING PROGRAMS

The Cognitive Sphere

How do socialization processes in the various nursing programs differ according to the cognitive abilities of their students? Little direct research has been done on this subject, but differences in socialization can be conjectured from Wren's descriptions of prototypical students.

It is generally assumed in academia that if students have sufficient intelligence to complete the program, they will complete the program; and the more intelligent the student, the more likely the student is to complete the program. Wren's prototypical baccalaureate student scores higher than diploma and A.D. students on academic indicators, and it is generally assumed that graduates of baccalaureate programs are superior to other nurses in their knowledge base and their ability to reason. There are two problems with this assumption: First, it is difficult to test because there is a base-level control on the amount of knowledge that must be learned and retained to become a practicing nurse. All three types of students will take the same licensure exams. Second, the data on attrition in nursing make it apparent that there are factors involved in success other than intellectual ability. B.S.N. students show greater attrition rates than those in the other programs. Bayer and Schoenfeldt (1970) found that the actual risk of failure was less in A.D. than in baccalaureate programs. In 1966, more than 75% of those in A.D. programs graduated, compared with 72% from diploma programs and 61% from baccalaureate programs.

The attrition rate in the baccalaureate program could be a result of the socialization process. There is no indication that because entering students are brighter, more of them will become confident and capable practitioners. (In fact, there is no guarantee that they will become practitioners at all.) To put knowledge into effect, nurses must perceive themselves as confident, professional, and capable of performing tasks assigned to them. This confidence does not come from intellectual ability but from educational experiences that provide the basis for professional socialization.

Alutto and others (1971) report that nurses graduating from the different programs are similar in terms of their cognitive commitment to the nursing profession. This finding is more significant than the cognitive abilities of the entering freshmen, because the degree of commitment has a greater affect on the attrition rate.

In short, the research into this problem indicates that the result of the socialization process does not differ among programs even though there are striking differences in the intellectual aptitude of the students.

The Interactional Sphere

Development in this sphere is a result of interaction between the socializers and the students. Students bring various roles to the program. B.S.N. students are more likely to be upper-middle class than students in the other two programs; A.D. students are lower-middle class and are more likely to have to integrate the roles of wife and mother into the student role.

How will these differences affect the socializers? How will the faculty respond to the older woman trying to integrate a role of mother and wife into the nursing role? How does social class affect the expectations of faculty members? From what socioeconomic class are faculty members likely to come? Wren's (1971) study suggests that the faculty most likely comes from the upper-middle class. It is interesting to speculate what affect this has on diploma and A.D. students from lower socioeconomic strata.

Much of what can be said about the interaction of faculty and students must be conjecture. The research that has been done concerns students, is contradictory, and does not consider the large variation within groups. There is little research on nursing faculty. The affect of faculty norms, values, personality traits, and demographic characteristics on the student socialization process has never been considered. Research in sociology has shown that leadership and nonauthoritarian attitudes are related to social class; that is, upper-middle class people tend to be less authoritarian and more confident of their leadership ability (McKee, 1962). Among grammar school students, social standing is related to popularity, and middle class children are more likely to be picked as friends (Neugarten, 1946). Further, there is an indication that all individuals are more likely to identify with members of their own or higher social status groups (McKee, 1969). Individuals rarely look down socioeconomically to admire people or choose friends.

These sociological findings indicate that baccalaureate instructors are more comfortable with and trusting of their baccalaureate students. Conversely, the baccalaureate students are expected to reciprocate because the instructors represent individuals of their own social status group who became professional and can serve as good role models. The finding (Alutto and others, 1971) that the baccalaureate students are more homogeneous in their value system and higher in their level of trust substantiates this inference. The baccalaureate faculty is less authoritarian than either of the other two programs' faculties.

The first stage of compliance and its accompanying dependency is easier for students from baccalaureate programs, in which the students' latent identities match those of the instructors. Does this mean that they are more "professional" upon graduation than are students in the other programs? Research by Richards (1972) and Alutto and others (1971) indicates that B.S.N. students do in fact have a more "professional" set of values and attitudes. B.S.N. students expect to take responsibility for entire tasks and many aspects of patient care, whereas students from the other types of programs are less likely to think this way.

These researchers also found that B.S.N. students anticipated role conflict between the bureaucratic structure and their attempt to put into practice their conception of nursing. What Kramer (1974) found probably should not be called "reality shock." Students were not shocked by what they found in the first year. They encountered problems that the faculty had warned them about. What appears to be reality shock to the B.S.N. may be a reaction to the lack of theory that would help students cope with bureaucratic problems. In any case, B.S.N. students' anticipation of the type of conflicts that induce many to leave the field (sometimes for teaching) indicates that baccalaureate students have indeed identified with their instructors. In fact, they have identified to the point that they see themselves following in the path their instructors have laid down for them and upon graduation, when faced with the same problems described by the role models, leave hospital nursing.

Alutto and others (1971) found that baccalaureate nurses do not demonstrate an ability to adjust to or cope with confrontation between bureaucratic and professional ideals. This indicates that, although trust and compliance may be easier for B.S.N. students, there is no evidence that constructive rebellion is encouraged in baccalaureate programs any more than it is in the other two programs. B.S.N. practitioners play their roles as programed by the socializers. They are told they will become uncomfortable upon graduation and experience role conflict. Upon graduation, they do in fact experience this. Their response is not to rebel. They internalize another set of values, eventually becoming disillusioned, or they leave the field (Corwin and others, 1961).

In contrast to this, diploma students are not likely to identify with the faculty and will not show the corresponding trust. They learn to exhibit the appropriate attitudes that allow them to fit into the hospital setting and survive. They experience less reality shock and remain in hospital nursing—often in the same hospital where they were trained. They are never as indoctrinated by the faculty as are B.S.N. students.

In spite of this, they have not reached Stage IV. They are still part of a culture that stresses obedience. They too need additional time after graduation to feel truly comfortable (Davis and others, 1966). They are, however, more comfortable with the hospital bureaucracy than the B.S.N. students are. They do not interpret the need to perform bureaucratic duties as necessarily forfeiting their professional responsibilities.

The Personality Sphere

Harry Stack Sullivan (1953) once observed that we are all more human than otherwise. The implication is that, because of human potential, similarities among individuals are as great as their differences. Although some researchers found differences in personality variables among students from the three different types of educational programs (Alutto, 1971; Meleis and Farrell, 1974), other researchers such as Richards (1972) found few differences. In fact, Meleis and Farrell were surprised by the amount of similarity among students in the various programs. One striking finding was the low self-esteem scores in the three schools — all were well below those of the normal college population. This finding reinforces the research cited in Chapter 6, which indicates that nurses have trouble accepting themselves and their impulses.

There is a great variance among diploma school students in personality factors on psychological tests (HEW report, 1975). When the 16 Personality Factor (16 P.F.) Questionnaire (Cattell, 1952) was analyzed, three major personality typologies emerged. Type I did not differ from the standard sample used for comparison, college women in general. Type I students exemplify Kardiner's (1945) "modal personality," whose personality patterns reflect the society as a whole, with its prevailing cultural mores, norms, and approved psychological defenses. Type II was the "neurotic introvert." These individuals tested high on the anxiety and neurotic defense mechanism scales, and scored low on the leadership scales. One subgroup within the type scored high in creativity, possibly indicating some outlet for the anxiety. Type III, "normal self-reliance," tested low on the anxiety neurosis and leadership scales, and high on the scale measuring alert poise. All three types did well in school and graduated. This study indicates that (a) normal women with test profiles resembling normal college students, (b) very neurotic women, and (c) women who are usually poised and self-reliant do well in nursing. Students who can trust their environment and get along in groups also do well.

What does this say about diploma students' progress through the stages of socialization? Those who are emotionally predisposed to trust and do well within a group (Stage I and III) are most likely to graduate. None of the traits that demand autonomy and initiative (Stage II) showed up as predictors for successful programs completion. Even the "self-reliant" students tested low on leadership, which indicates a certain lack of initiative.

These findings about the significant personality traits that correlate with success in diploma school education may help explain the disparity in the results of the various studies. The differences found between entering students and students still in school do not seem to affect the finished product. Students from the different programs may vary along such dimensions as age, socioeconomic status, and perhaps (although here there is much dissention) aptitude. However, upon graduation all these students have the same status attained by licensure and encounter similar problems. What the baccalaureate program accomplishes in the selection process with its expanded and expensive curriculum, the diploma schools apparently accomplish through the socialization process that provides for personality traits screening. Baccalaureate students are better off in Stage I because their higher socioeconomic status makes it easier for them to trust the socializers. In diploma schools, those students whose personality dynamics predispose them to trust are more likely to graduate. The older A.D. student is less dependent upon the socializers; in this program, trust is not as much an issue within the educational process.

In one sense, then, the process of socialization can be said to work in similar ways in all programs. Students are selected because they are most likely to meet faculty expectations and to get along well with their peers. None of the faculties expect or demand autonomy and initiative—they expect to be agreed with, even to the extent that students identify with their professional problems. The idea that "a nurse is a nurse is a nurse" may not be true, but nursing students appear to be (to paraphrase Sullivan) "more nurses than otherwise."

DOES RESISTANCE EXIST IN NURSING EDUCATION?

A major contention of Chapter 4 was that the structure of nursing education supports dependent behavior characteristics of Stage I in all three spheres. There is evidence in the literature that Stage II (resistance) would be difficult for students in any of the nursing programs.

These assertions cannot be studied directly. No empirical research has been done in this area, and there are no tests devised specifically to test these hypotheses. However, the studies that measure attitude changes in nursing students from their entrance into nursing education to graduation can be analyzed to see whether the students are progressing through the stages of socialization. This will be done by focusing on the changes found in personality traits and values over time and the different ways students in the three programs experience these changes.

Again, a caveat about these studies: While there are many studies of nursing students, only a few of the studies have been longitudinal. Most compare a group of seniors with a group of freshmen tested at the same time, and thus present serious problems in interpretation. They make an assumption that cannot be checked: the research is based on the premise that current seniors entered with the same characteristics that the current freshmen now show. Comparison of 18-year-old freshmen with 21-year-old seniors could show differences in personality characteristics, values, and identities as a function of the maturation process alone and not reflect the educational socialization process. Despite the problems of interpretation, these studies provide the only evidence indicating the changes nursing students undergo during their socialization.

Cognitive Changes

The conventional examination and grading system provides a continuous assessment of the knowledge base as students progress through nursing education. But few studies concern themselves with the processes of problem-solving and whether these thought processes change over time. Most studies correlate academic predictor scores and high school grades to success in nursing.

The exceptions to this rule are the studies done on creativity. Creativity can be seen as an indicator that students have experienced Stage II (resistance) and have tried out alternatives rather than learning one right answer. The instruments used to study creativity emphasize multiple interpretations of the same object and indicate an ability to examine the situation from several points of view and to recognize the existence of several viable solutions. Students who can do this presumably are no longer in Stage I (dependency), simply absorbing the intellectual content from their instructors. They examine content, think of other alternatives, and check out these alternatives with their classmates.

Are students more creative when they graduate from nursing school than they are when they enter? The literature on creativity and nursing students is sparse and conflicting. Torrance (1964) studied two successive classes and found them to be more creative in their senior year than in their freshman year. Eisenman (1970), using the same instruments as Torrance and including cross-sectional and longitudinal data, found a decrease in originality. Why these conflicting results? An examination of Torrance's study shows that test/retest learning and practice may have affected the results, and the experimentor may have biased the results of the study. Torrance administered the test to the students in her psychiatric nursing course and insisted that they practice beforehand; that is, the students were taught how to give alternative forms and answers to many types of questions. Eisenman, on the other hand, carefully controlled for the learning effect with alternative forms and by gathering the sample from many classes in different schools.

Torrance's results could be interpreted as showing that the students became more dependent rather than more creative. When their instructor insisted that they be creative and give alternative responses, they did so, but it was a rote-learned response. This has nothing to do with resisting the instructors' interpretation of material or with establishing mutuality with classmates to learn to utilize different approaches in different situations. Eisenman's study indicates that nursing education precludes this process.

Changes in the Interactional Sphere

Studies that measure changes in students' values and attitudes can indicate how far students have progressed in the interactional sphere. However, it is not enough for the students to have changed. The goal in the interactional sphere is the integration of personal norms and values with those of the profession. Progression through the stages might be measured by two factors. The first is how much a student's values and attitudes have become like those considered acceptable by the profession. The second is the degree to which these new values and attitudes have been incorporated into the student's own values.

If students' values, attitudes, and image of the profession do not change but continue to resemble those held by lay people, they have not yet begun the process of socialization. When students begin Stage I they hold the values of lay people, and in the socialization process they move toward the values held by their instructors. In Stage II, students should question the values in the field. Students in Stage III should begin to espouse their instructors' view of the field and professional values and attitudes, but since this is the stage of experimentation their values and images in the field have not jelled. Only during Stage IV should a set of values and images of the role in the field be solidified and internalized into the student's personal set of values.

In reality, do students follow this pattern of socialization? Research on changes in attitudes and values over time indicates that seniors do exhibit some Stage III characteristics. But there is also evidence that they have not totally discarded their pre-Stage I values and attitudes. It is apparent in most of the studies that values and attitudes do not change very much between the freshman and the senior years. Indeed, Olesen and Davis (1966), in their study of baccalaureate students, were surprised at how little change had taken place between freshmen and seniors. Sharp and Anderson (1972) also found only small differences between beginning and graduating baccalaureate students.

This does not mean that there were no differences between freshmen and seniors. While senior baccalaureate students retained many of the stereotypes about nursing that they had had when they entered nursing school, they did add a professional quality to their image of the nursing field. The students' professional values were inconsistent, and included some ambivalence (Sharp and Anderson, 1972). This is characteristic of Stage II (resistance).

Senior students exhibited Stage III characteristics by not having a consensus on what nursing was really like. Fewer graduating students than entering students agreed on an image of nursing. As freshmen, they apparently shared strong and consistent images of the role propounded by the culture and carried by the media; upon graduation, they disagreed on what nursing was really about (Sharp and Anderson, 1972). These findings conform to our model, which predicts that in Stage III students experiment and choose aspects of the role that are most important to them personally, as well as being professionally acceptable.

Internalization of the ideologies and a conception of the role common to the entire field are characteristic of Stage IV. Sharp and Anderson (1972) ran an item analysis and found that on those items on which differences between seniors and freshmen existed, the seniors more nearly resembled the faculty than did the freshmen. However, on the test as a whole, seniors still differed significantly from the faculty. Although seniors were beginning to view the field as their instructors did, they did not yet share their instructors' image of nursing. This would indicate that seniors have not yet resolved Stage III.

Do entering students view nursing differently than graduating students and practitioners? Many studies have indicated that nursing students enter nursing because they want to help people (McDonald, 1969; Katz and Martin, 1972; Barnartt and Cohen, 1976). Meyer (1960) studied students in the three different types of educational programs and found that upon graduation the students had discarded their initial view of the nurse as a ministering angel. Understandably, the entering freshmen would espouse the cultural stereotype of the nursing role. At the end of their education, most students had expanded the role to include more of the professional, knowledgeable, and objective qualities. This change was less apparent in A.D. students. However, students from all programs were technically and emotionally oriented to patient care, and were aware that there could be negative outcomes regardless of their best efforts.

Several studies document a similar change in a generally benevolent attitude toward the world and a desire to help people, usually designated as humanitarianism. Both Eron (1955) and Moody (1973) found that entering freshmen are much more humanitarian than are seniors, who are more cynical. Psathas (1969) found senior diploma students to be less idealistic and more pessimistic than their freshman counterparts.

These changes from the humanitarian to the more cynical and pessimistic and less idealistic have sometimes dismayed nursing educators. This dismay is probably caused by the semantics of the description rather than the actual attitude of the students. An examination of the various scales used to measure humanitarianism indicates that the seniors receive lower scores because they substitute a professionally useful, pragmatic attitude for the highly idealized lay attitude with which they enter the profession. As Psathas states:

> The realism, and what sometimes appears to be cynicism concerning the nurse's tasks and duties and her interaction with patients, doctors and nurses, represents an awareness of events that can and do occur in the situations depicted. The senior responses show that situations that were formerly difficult and disturbing or were described as containing considerable diversity of activity, become routine, understandable and easily dealt with.*

Williams and Williams (1959) looked at how students manage to cope with those aspects of nursing judged by society to be dirty, disgusting, or untouchable. They found that students substituted for lay attitudes the values of selflessness, untiring service, and scientific cause and effect. Without these professional values they would have had difficulty working successfully in their role. Williams and Williams do not necessarily indicate that students' progression through the stages proposed here is a prerequisite to becoming independent practitioners. The students may have been merely adopting and

*From Psathas, G. 1969. The fate of idealism in nursing schools. *Journal of Health and Social Behavior* 9:87.

trusting their instructors' attitudes in these areas without either resisting or trying to look for alternatives.

It is difficult to tell from these studies whether the students were in Stage I or Stage III in the interactional sphere. There indeed had been change. Their values are not the same as the values with which they entered nursing school. There is, however, no indication that they took part in any type of Stage II resistance. Their values more nearly resembled those that were acceptable for the field. The students did not move away from the professional values; they moved toward what had been presented to them as acceptable. The senior students were successsful in the program because they had managed to conform to the faculty's expectations.

Changes in the Personality Sphere

Changes in the personality sphere are not easily measured. Few of the commonly used personality tests have factors that specifically relate to trust, autonomy, industry, or identity. However, what is striking about the studies that do attempt to assess personality changes over the years needed to complete the educational process is that few changes are found. This is true regardless of the type of instrument used in the testing (Redden and Scales, 1961; Mitchell, 1977).

A literature search reveals a dearth of research on personality changes in nursing students from freshman to senior year. There are, however, many studies that address the problems of integrating the professional role and the female sex role. (See Chapter 7 for a discussion of nursing as a female occupation.) This is a Stage III problem: Can the individual integrate the professional concepts necessary to become a nurse and also maintain a satisfactory sexual identity?

Stromberg (1976) points out that the traditional female personality traits do not include independence, leadership, competence, or intellectual achievement. Therefore, changes in the student's sexual identity would be necessary to integrate the "professional nurse" and the female self-perception. Stromberg also found that students with more masculine sex role identities held images of nursing resembling those of practicing nurses. Students whose sex role identities were more traditionally feminine did not.

Another study (Levitt and others, 1962) compared sophomore (preclinical) baccalaureate students with graduate nurses. In their results the preclinical students were much more feminine. They were characterized as nurturant, deferential, and lacking aggressiveness, autonomy, and dominance. The graduate nurses were much more masculine on everything except autonomy.

Stage IV integration is based on successful Stage II resistance. The graduate, if she continues in the field, must at some point experience resistance and interdependence on her way to independence. There is no indication this is encouraged or even allowed in nursing schools.

In a longitudinal study (HEW Grant, 1975), the Henry and Sims (1970) Identity Scale was administered to four classes of diploma students. This scale consists of six dimensions involved in an individual's decision about his or her identity:

1. Identity:
   a. Career
   b. Group membership
   c. Evaluation of self
   d. Positive effectual experience
2. Expressivity and comfort with the social contacts
3. Individualistic expressivity
4. Integrity
5. Autonomy within social limits
6. Trust

The tests were given under two different sets of instructions. The first had students describe their self-identity—that is, "myself as I really am." The second had students describe the "ideal nurse." The "ideal nurse" presumably represented the students' professional goal; the "myself as I really am" indicated the students' present identity. Correlations between the real identity and the professional goal at the beginning of the freshman and at the end of the senior year are presented in Table 5–1.

When students enter nursing school, there is a strong relationship between their self-perception and their professional ideal in the areas of trust, autonomy, and identity. Students apparently come into nursing holding stereotypes about the field consonant with their perceived identities. High correlations probably reflect an interactional process in which students alter their self-perceptions to fit the nursing role, and modify their stereotypes to fit their self-perceptions.

The correlations for students approaching graduation looked quite different. There is still a positive relationship between their perceived identity and their professional ideal, but the relationships are not as strong. The lower cor-

TABLE 5-1   Correlations Between Present Identity and Professional Ideal

	Freshman year N = 106	Senior year N = 106
Trust	r = .44**	r = .21*
Autonomy	r = .41**	r = .03 N.S.
Identity	r = .34**	r = .20*

Note: The factor scores were computed from individual items on the Sims (1962) Identity Scale.
  * $p = .01$
** $p = .001$

relations in the senior year suggest that the students' personalities have been strongly affected by the socialization process. Most notable is the autonomy factor: There is virtually no relationship between the amount of autonomy the student describes herself as having and the amount of autonomy she thinks the ideal nurse should have. The students obviously believe that the degree of autonomy that they experience has no relationship to the autonomy that characterizes their professional ideal. This negligible correlation seems to indicate that students have not yet begun to resolve their feeling about autonomy. Stage II concerns are clearly problems for senior nursing students because they cannot see how their self-perceptions and their professional goals can be integrated.

Although the correlations in the trust and identity factors have also fallen, the correspondence between the perception of self and the perception of the idealized nurse is still significant. Lower correlations indicate that the students have made some progress in professional socialization. They are no longer relying upon the stereotypes of the field or upon the values of the instructors. However, the fact that the correlations are still significant indicates that these students are still very concerned with Stage I types of problems and solutions. Indeed, it may indicate that they view trusting as an integral component of the nursing role. There is nothing wrong with trust, but if the trust is an indication of the dependency of Stage I and the corresponding problems, then clearly these students are not professionally socialized.

Evidence that Student
Resistance (Stage II) Does Exist

Despite the concern of seniors about autonomy and the indication that there are few changes in values between freshman and senior years, the literature does contain descriptions of student reactions that could be categorized as resistance. One manifestation of resistance is a refusal to give up values under faculty pressure. Davis and Olesen (1963) identified a grief reaction in students 3 months after they entered the nursing part of a baccalaureate program. The students voiced objections toward the perceived lack of femininity demanded by the nursing role. They felt that in learning this new role they would have to give up a treasured part of their old feminine identities. Their response to this demand was to devalue the nursing role. In this way they justified maintaining their prized femininity in the face of faculty disapproval.

In a subsequent paper (1964) Davis and Olesen identified several more profession-specific types of resistance. During the first year, the students retained many elements of the lay image of nursing, despite faculty preference for a more professional image. The students also resisted the faculty's claim that the content of nursing theory was "solid intellectual content" and were less prone to believe that nursing was a well-respected occupation. Two years later this resistance was not diminishing significantly. Resistance did not take the form of overt rebellion. It was passive resistance, consisting of clinging to stereotypes and an unwillingness to accept instructors' values.

In Brown and others' (1974) replication of the Davis and Olesen study, the same kinds of resistance were found. Juniors were less likely to believe the professional image of nursing propounded by the instructors than were sophomores. Again, resistance was subtle but present. Meyer (1960) also found that lay stereotypes of the field were not easily given up by students. In this sample, the greatest resistance was to be found in the A.D. schools.

Resistance does not only manifest itself in opposition to the faculty's image of nursing; it also takes an emotional form. Ingmire (1959) found that first-year students were quite happy in school. Second-year students, however, were highly sensitive, with easily hurt feelings, and felt inferior to other students. Their reactions were in general much less positive than those of the first-year students, and they seemed critical of almost every facet of their education. Third-year students had dissatisfactions but these were focused on their team role. The results of this study would indicate that second-year students were going through Stage II and finding it difficult. The third-year students would be coping with Stage III issues, a period during which students are not critical of everything but focus on the role problems and group processes. They were apparently attempting to construct a role identity that would make sense to them.

The strongest evidence for the existence of Stage II in any nursing education program comes from Olesen and Whittaker's (1968) book on a baccalaureate nursing school. They found evidence of what they called "studentsmanship," which "functions to suggest answers to a perpetually problematic issue: how to get through school with the greatest comfort and the least effort, preserving oneself as a person, while at the same time being a success and attaining the necessities for one's future life." Studentsmanship is nothing less than a student culture, dedicated to getting through and attaining the degree while maintaining the sense of self—in this case, femininity. Student cultures provide group vehicles for Stage II, but they cannot easily be observed, nor do they reveal themselves on psychological tests with pre-set answers. An observational study conducted by Olesen and Whittaker demonstrated that, despite the kind of repression that existed, students developed strategies for getting through and held values that did not match the values of their faculty.

The medical students studied by Becker (1961) were much more explicit in their circumvention of the system. They divided up material, tried to "psych out" what would be on the examinations, and studied as little as possible. They felt no need to con the faculty or present themselves as scholars. The medical faculty neither knew nor cared about this attitude until the research report detailing the phenomenon was published. Nursing students under closer faculty surveillance would be more careful in developing such a study scheme.

They must not only pass examinations — they must also always look bright and alert both to their nursing faculty and the staff on the wards.

The studies by Olesen and associates show that resistance does take place in the interactional sphere. My testing of diploma students indicates that nursing students are very concerned with autonomy. Research on nursing does not support the notion that Stage II is nonexistent, but it does indicate that the manifestations of Stage II are usually "passive aggressive." In other words, students do resist but they do not wish to be caught doing it, and therefore, resistant behavior is very difficult to isolate.

A Compounding Problem

Nursing students have many problems with feeling professional at graduation. They have difficulty expressing Stage II resistance, and stages in the different spheres are not synchronized so that learning in one can be reinforced by others. At graduation they are still in Stage I in the cognitive sphere and struggling with the tasks of Stages II and III in the interactional and personality spheres.

This asynchrony makes it more difficult for students to resolve the stages, and the result is no resolution. Dependence lingers on throughout the formal socialization process. Stage II, predictably, crops up in subtle ways, since open expression of resistance is not sanctioned.

This confusion of stages is compounded by the fact that students are not expected nor encouraged by their instructors to reach Stage IV before graduation. Students do not graduate ready for independent action or for continued commitment to their profession. They have not developed an acceptable role identity as professionals. Their identities and professional roles do not mesh, so they are not attached to their role.

If students are to be successful in their professional role, socialization must continue until they have resolved Stage IV. But as Kramer (1974) notes, on-the-job socialization in a hospital is a precarious and doubtful occurrence. Socialization is in the hands of physicians, staff nurses, and sometimes aides. What the new graduate learns depends on the milieu of the first job. The profession makes no systematic attempt to continue the socialization process, but leaves the new graduate floundering. It is not surprising that Kramer found them susceptible to professional disillusionment. In fact, it is perfectly consistent with, and predictable from, the evidence reviewed in this chapter.

Part III

SPECIFIC PROBLEMS
IN NURSING EDUCATION

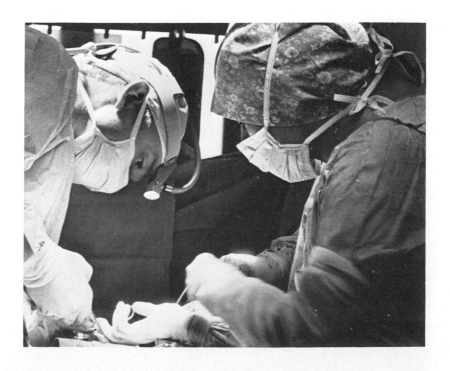

Chapter 6

PERSONALITY FACTORS

Although research on nursing has not focused on the cognitive or psychological components of the professional socialization process, the problem of attrition has been studied extensively. The nursing attrition rate, which ranges from 30% to 50%, has been of much concern to educators and researchers alike. Knopf (1975) indicates that nursing attrition is more expensive and harmful to nursing education than to a college program because nursing schools usually do not have flexible curricula. Students who enter together become a class going through the same educational experiences at the same time. If a course is not completed satisfactorily, a student cannot take it over again the next semester; she must wait and reenter with the next class. A student who drops out of school or fails one segment is a student lost to that graduating class. There is no way to catch up during the summer. (Recent changes in curriculum and the success of self-pacing programs may solve this problem.)

Studies on attrition have focused on the cognitive abilities and personalities of nursing students. A review of the research on nursing students' personality characteristics is pertinent to an analysis of the socialization process because it provides evidence that Stage II, resistance, is discouraged by the educational system in nursing. Studies indicate that nursing students share certain personality characteristics, such as submissiveness and dependency, which generally preclude an active and resistive personality. This chapter examines work done on personality and attrition in nursing students and presents the results of my research on personality patterns of successful nursing students. Finally, some recent developments are analyzed for signs of a changing nursing personality. (How the educational system specifically encourages dependency was discussed in Part II.)

STUDIES ON ATTRITION IN NURSING

Standard Tests

Cognitive factors were the first and most prominent issue investigated by researchers interested in attrition. Cognitive factors were correlated with success in nursing education to establish objective predictive entrance exams.

Many investigators have noted the predictive power of cognitive factors (Ford, 1950; French, 1961; and Murphy, 1965). However, the predictive power of cognitive tests depends on the criteria used. Munday and Hoyt (1956) studied seven nursing schools in the South and Midwest with a total of 1513 first-year students and found the ACT to be an excellent predictor of academic success (0.7 or higher correlation with first year grades). However, Munday and Hoyt concluded that a major drawback of the study was the various standards of excellence represented by the seven schools. The grading procedures ranged from difficult to easy. These differences among the groups were reflected in the ACT data and, as a result, generalization of the predictive power of the ACT is hazardous despite the high correlation.

Plapp and others (1966) found that complex motivational and personal factors replaced intellectual factors as the major reasons for attrition after the first year.

Gerstein (1965) investigated the use of multiple choice tests as a selection device for females entering a 3-year nursing education program. The subjects for this study were 29 students in the class of 1962 and 42 students in the class of 1963. Prior to their acceptance into the program, all students were given the Otis Self-Administering Test of Mental Ability, the IPAT Culture Free Test (g), the Diagnostic Reading Survey (Form C), and the Strong Vocational Interest Test. Three years later, on the basis of these measures, the graduating students were compared to those students who did not complete the program. Significant differences between graduates and withdrawals were found only on the Diagnostic Reading Surveys. Prediction of success or failure based upon cut-off scores was accurate in 78% to 87% of the cases for both withdrawals and graduates.

May (1966) emphasizes the importance of nonintellectual factors for predicting success, after finding that dropouts scored higher on the theoretical and economic portions of the Allport-Vernon study of values. Those who stayed in school scored higher on the social scale.

From this it becomes apparent that, although intellectual factors play an important role in the student's ability to complete a nursing education program, it is unquestionably not the only factor. Indeed, among students who have the intellectual capacity to complete a program, personality factors appear to be the crucial variable in determining their success in school. We will now review research substantiating this theory.

The most comprehensive investigation dealing with the causes of student attrition in nursing education was done by Teal and Fabrizio (1961). Through personal interviews, background data (entrance examination results, high school records, and IQ) were obtained from 269 dropouts and 387 continuing students from 12 schools of nursing. All subjects were given student questionnaires. Teal and Fabrizio (1961) report a close relationship between the mental ability characteristics of the nonacademic dropout and the continuing student. The nonacademic dropout and the continuing student generally stood higher in their high school graduating classes than did the academic dropout. Intelligence tests scores of nonacademic dropouts and continuing students were similar, and were generally higher than those of academic dropouts. Further, Teal and Fabrizio reported a good number of emotional reasons for both types of withdrawals, and concluded that many cases probably could have been salvaged had counseling services outside of the instructor and disciplinary chain been available. The authors then rank-ordered the ten most frequently stated reasons for withdrawals given by academic and nonacademic dropouts. Table 6-1 summarizes their findings.

TABLE 6-1   Reasons for Withdrawal in Schools of Nursing with Rank Orders
            Given by Academic and Nonacademic Dropouts

Rank	Reasons given by academic dropouts	Reasons given by nonacademic dropouts
1	Near or actual failure	Marriage and/or pregnancy
2	Did not know how to study	Lost interest in nursing
3	Pressure and tension in school created emotional strain	Pressure and tension in school created emotional strain
4	Tried hard, but could not grasp material	Personal problems interfered with education
5	Became fatigued, depressed, nervous, and could not sleep	Disappointed in nursing school; it did not match expectations
6	Not enough preparation in subject matter prior to nursing school	Did not receive enough satisfaction from giving nursing care
7	Living conditions (noise in dormitory, roommate, conditions at home, etc.) interfered with studying	Became fatigued, depressed, nervous, and could not sleep
8	Did not put enough time and effort into studying	Decided that the hours, pay, and working conditions of the R.N. were not what I wanted in the future
9	Nursing school staff did not appear interested in whether students stayed	Curriculum was not broad enough; did not include enough subjects other than nursing
10	Not enough clinical experience	Did not like the way most courses were taught

Cohen, H.A. (principal investigator). 1975a. Review of literature section. HEW Report 05000309 04NOO10.

Interestingly, both academic and nonacademic dropouts complained that the pressure and tension in the school created emotional strain and that there were problems with the educational system. The nonacademic dropouts did not like the way the courses were taught; the academic dropouts felt the nursing school staff did not appear interested in whether students stayed. Teal and Fabrizio did not probe to find out what students found disappointing in nursing (either with the educational system or with nursing care), why students thought the curriculum was not broad enough, or what students did not like about their courses.

It is surprising that investigation of these issues has been so general and not focused on the exact problems and emotional causes of attrition in nursing education. In 1975, Knopf reported the results of the Nurse Career Pattern study. This study, initiated by the National League of Nursing, is a longitudinal study designed to obtain definitive information on nursing students. It investigates students' biographical characteristics, occupational goals, reasons for choosing a career in nursing, and contribution to the health field after graduation. After examining the reasons for withdrawal from nursing school, Knopf came to the following conclusion: "It is apparent that among baccalaureate programs and, to a lesser extent among the associate degree programs, directors of the nursing programs were unaware of the reasons why students left nursing school." The literature, instead of focusing on the problems students experience with the educational system or with the faculty, had analyzed the personality factors of the successful nursing student and the successful practitioner.

Many early studies utilizing the Minnesota Multi-phasic Personality Inventory (MMPI) (Benett and Gordon, 1944; Spaney, 1953; Thurston, Brunclick, and Feldhusen, 1969) failed to differentiate the successful nursing students from the unsuccessful ones or the nursing student from the normal college student. Wersgerber (1954) established scale norms for the MMPI with nursing students. He tested 168 student nurses in the Chicago area and found nursing students to have stable, normal personality characteristics. However, in 1957 Wersgerber attempted to correlate the MMPI variables with ratings on 19 personality traits rated necessary for good student nursing by a sample of nursing educators, and found trends but no significant correlations between practical ratings and MMPI. Overall, Wersgerber concluded that the MMPI is not a useful predictor of training aptitude and occupational fitness.

Researchers tried to factor the MMPI to find items that discriminated between groups of college women and nursing students. Beaver (1953), utilizing this technique, found 65 items that discriminated at the 0.05 level of significance between education majors and nursing students. The 65 items were grouped into four categories: "social sexual factors," "adherence to customs," "psychosomatic concerns," and "freedom from neuroticism." Beaver found that nursing students preferred their own sex, liked tall masculine women, and did not find pleasure in social dancing. They were prudish in attitude, embarrassed by dirty stories, and tended to avoid sexy shows. They disapproved of women smoking and drinking alcoholic beverages and considered duty as life's goal. They did not worry much about their health and seldom played sick. In the last category, "freedom from neuroticism," nursing students were found to be stable. They denied fears of people or dark places, and anxiety and tensions were not part of their life.

Malher (1955) tried to verify Beaver's study and found that only 13 of the 65 items discriminated between nursing and nonnursing students. Indeed, he concluded that, contrary to Beaver's findings, there was little difference between nursing students and college women as measured by the MMPI or by the specific item analysis.

Researchers then began to substitute the Edwards' Personal Preference Schedule (EPPS) for the MMPI. This was accelerated after Navran and Stauffacher (1957) noted that most studies with the MMPI and with other inventories had found few significant correlations. Navran and Stauffacher thought that the EPPS was superior to previous inventories because the way the questions were stated corrected for the susceptibility of the inventories to subjects' faking or manipulation by the investigator. The remainder of this section examines the results from researchers utilizing the EPPS as their instrument.

Redden and Scales (1961) used the EPPS to compare nursing students with college women. They found significant differences on 12 of the 15 variables. Nursing students scored higher in deference, introception, nurturance, endurance, and aggression; and lower in order, exhibition, autonomy, affiliation change, dominance, and heterosexuality.

Reece (1961) attempted to assess personality characteristics associated with success in a nursing program. A sample of 87 female nursing students was divided into two groups, successful and unsuccessful. (Success was defined as graduation from the program.) The two groups were compared to the sample on which this test was standardized. The successful nursing students were more submissive, deferent, persistent, and nurturant than college women in general. They had less need to achieve and to dominate others. In comparing the unsuccessful group with college women in general, Reece summarizes:

> In general, the profile for the Withdrawal group falls between the Completed and the norm groups. These students tend to be more like the norm subjects in the needs for achievement, deference, order, endurance, and aggression. On the other hand they tend more toward the Completed group in autonomy, succorance, abasement, change, and heterosexuality. The scores for exhibition, dominance, and nurturance fell almost in the middle, between the norm and completed groups.*

Levitt and others (1962) compared 212 freshman nursing students with

*From Reece, M.M. 1961. Personality characteristics and success in a nursing program. *Nursing Research* 10(3):175.

Edwards' 749 college women in general, and found differences on eight of the 15 variables. Nursing students were higher on the variables of order, succorance, nurturance, and abasement, and lower on achievement, autonomy, dominance, and aggression. Levitt suggests that the data indicate a preclinical personality pattern for nursing students that emphasizes feminine needs, while assertive needs are played down.

Caputo and Hanf (1965) undertook a comprehensive comparison of various groups to test the existence of an occupational personality in nursing. Compared on the EPPS were two groups of R.N.'s, two groups of senior nursing students, two groups of freshman nursing students, one group of college women, one group of adult women, and one group of high school graduates. The groups correlated significantly with each other on all scales. R.N.'s correlated significantly with each other, with nursing students, and also with adult women and college women. Senior and freshman nursing students correlated highly with each other and also with high school graduates and college women. Caputo and Hanf summarize their results:

> In general, rank-order correlation methods appear to demonstrate that, although there is a communality of personality attitudes as measured by the EPPS among most nursing groups, these groups are not consistently discriminated from other groups of females who are not involved in nursing.*

In attempting to explain the results, Caputo and Hanf suggest that nursing is an expedient way of obtaining financial security and independence prior to marriage, and that personality needs may not be influential in an individual's choosing nursing. They cite Habenstein and Christ (1955), who implied that occupational testing should be administered only to those who remain active in and are heavily committed to the field. Caputo and Hanf also state that nursing is too diverse to use a broad vocational designation and that specific dimensions or tasks require further research.

Casella (1968) attempted to replicate Caputo and Hanf's study after finding methodological errors in their comparison of the different groups. Casella administered the EPPS to 97 female nursing students. The comparison group consisted of 125 liberal arts college women. Direct comparison of the two groups by test failed to yield any significant differences on the 15 variables. The profiles were ranked and compared by means of the Spearman Rank Order correlation and were significantly related at the 0.05 level. Casella summarized the results:

> It appears more prudent and empirically valid to say that the EPPS, based on the samples tested, failed to provide a legitimate basis for discrimination

*From Caputo, V., and Hanf, C. 1965. EPPS patterns and the nursing personality. *Educational and Psychological Measures* 25:432.

between nursing students and nonnurses. Their need profiles, being interrelated, appear to be relatively homogeneous.*

In "Comparative Analysis of Personality Structure of Nursing Students," Bailey and Claus (1969) used the EPPS to test three hypotheses. To investigate whether a certain type of personality enters nursing, they compared four successive sophomore classes at the University of California from 1965 to 1969. Second, the authors compared these four classes with Edwards' college women in general to test the distinctiveness of nursing students. Finally, the University of California nursing students were compared with samples from Wayne State University and Indiana University to see if a homogeneous pattern holds up in different institutions.

The four successive classes of sophomores were similar, with a difference only on the variable of aggression. In comparing the four classes with college women in general, 11 significant differences were found: nursing students scored higher on the needs deference, introception, nurturance, and endurance, and lower on exhibition, autonomy, succorance, dominance, change, heterosexuality, and aggression. Bailey and Claus explain the nursing student's need pattern:

> . . . to find out what others think and want (deference), to be sensitive to others' feelings (introception), to be kind, sympathetic, and helpful (nurturance), and to work hard at and complete a job (endurance). That this and other nursing student groups differ from a general sample of college women is also clear, the latter being characterized as more dominant and aggressive.**

A great deal of similarity was found between nursing students of different institutions. There were, however, some differences among institutions on a number of variables. These differences may be the result of different programs and locations. Despite the differences, a pattern emerges in rank-ordering. Bailey and Claus describe the student nurses as "conforming to custom, being orderly, analytical of human behavior, abasing, having a high degree of persistence on a task, and above all being nurturant."

Adams and Klein (1970) noted the diversity in the literature comparing the nurse and/or nursing student with contrasting groups. They hypothesize that temporal factors account for the lack of agreement concerning the personality of the nursing student. They suggest that the EPPS may be sensitive to broad changes across generations of nurses. To test their hypothesis, Adams and Klein compared 50 nursing students with Edwards' 1954 norms for college women, with Klein's 1957 sample of high school students, and with Gynther

*From Casella, C. 1968. Need hierarchies among nursing and nonnursing college students. *Nursing Research* 17:274.
**From Bailey, J.T., and Claus, K.E. 1969. Comparative analysis of the personality structure of nursing students. *Nursing Research* 18:323.

and Gertz's 1959 sample of nursing students who had graduated from the same high school.

In comparing the 1970 sample of nursing students with Edwards' sample of college women in general, nursing students were found to score significantly lower on deference, autonomy, and dominance, and significantly higher on abasement, nurturance, and heterosexuality. In comparison to Klein's high school sample, nursing students scored significantly lower on autonomy, exhibition, change, and aggression, and higher on introception and nurturance. Compared to Edwards' norms, the 1959 sample of nursing students of Gynther and Gertz scored higher on exhibition, autonomy, dominance, and change. The only finding that was replicated in the 1970 comparison of nursing students with Edwards' norms was nursing students' lower scores on autonomy. Adams and Klein conclude:

> The current groups of nursing students did not differ from the normative group on the need order or need endurance scale, representing a direct change not only from the findings of Gynther and Gertz but also from the majority of other findings in the literature. While these results are difficult to explain, they suggest a lessened concern among the current nursing student with routine, neatness, organization, persistence, and accomplishment, which can be said to parallel, if not necessarily to reflect, a larger trend among current college-age individuals.*

Findings by Bailey and Claus (1969), Levitt (1962), Reece (1961), and Redden and Scales (1961) indicate a pattern of needs for nursing students. All four studies show nursing students to be more deferent, nurturant, and enduring, and less dominant and autonomous than college women in general. Five other needs, however, were widely divergent. The research of Caputo and Hanf (1965), Casella (1968), and Adams and Klein (1970) indicates that nursing students are not significantly different from college women in general. While no two studies indicate total agreement on any need, five of the six studies show nurturance to be significantly higher and autonomy and dominance to be significantly lower in nursing students than in the comparison group.

Explanations for the Diverse Results   Adams and Klein suggest that the diversity in the literature may be related to temporal factors. Their findings show a change in nursing students in the 1970s, possibly reflective of a broad generational change. Klein had previously compared three successive sophomore classes with each other and found significant changes in successive classes. He found that there has been an increase in heterosexuality and autonomy in entering classes since 1962, coupled with a decrease in deference to authority and endurance. This tends to support Adams and Klein's hypothesis that there may be character changes taking place in nursing students as indi-

*From Adams, J., and Klein, L.R. 1970. Students in nursing school: Consideration in assessing personality characteristics. *Nursing Research* 19:364.

cated by an increase in autonomy and less concern with routine. Bailey and Claus' (1969) study is more congruent, however, with the previously cited studies of a decade ago than with the findings of Adams and Klein.

Methodological considerations may help explain the diversity of results. All of the studies used either a rank-order correlation or a *t* test to measure differences between the needs of nursing students and college women in general. No attempt was made to establish a complete picture of the nursing student either by measuring more than one dimension (need, values, IQ, etc.) or by understanding how the needs interrelate. It may be that rather than students entering nursing with one consistent need pattern, several patterns or styles exist. Some may be reflective of a changing society, while others may exhibit a need pattern congruent with the past generation.

Smith (1968) argued that motivation for nursing was complex and therefore, to understand the variance, more than one personality dimension must be assessed. Smith administered the EPPS and the Allport Vernon Study of Values to 546 freshman students from ten diploma schools in Baltimore. Using the rotated-factor matrix method, the 21 variables of the test were reduced to seven factors. The derived factors were:

> Factor I: Tender-hearted. This factor includes the need variables of affiliation, nurturance, and succorance, and the value, social. There is interest in establishing close connections and relations with others; relationships are characterized by loyalty, generosity, and a willingness to do things with and for others.
>
> Factor II: The strong-willed. Four variables—heterosexually, aggression, autonomy, and exhibition—have almost similar degrees of influence on this factor, while the fifth variable, succorance, has the least and is probably subsidiary to one or more of the variables of independence, self-determination and control, self-assertiveness, and confidence.
>
> Factor III: The religious-mystic. Three variables contribute to this dimension of personality. They are the values, religious and social, and the need, introception. Attitudes included in this group of variables are the realization of the deficiencies in existing social conditions from a humanistic standpoint; intuitive understanding of others free from judgments, and an interest in analyzing feelings, motives and behavior.
>
> Factor IV: The humble-religious. The need abasement and the social value have almost equal loading in this factor. They are accompanied by the value, religious, which has a decreased relative influence. The religious conviction arouses a reverence for life concomitant with attitudes of gratitude, humility, and a willingness to serve and obey.
>
> Factor V: The dependent-achiever. Of the four variables comprising this factor, the need succorance carries by far the most influence. The three remaining variables—achievement, order, and social—have smaller but comparable degrees of influence among themselves. In brief, this factor concerns active dependency coupled with the need to achieve, perhaps in a perfectionistic sense, with accompanying altruistic and philanthropic values.
>
> Factor VI: The intellectual-achiever. The value theoretic and the need achievement appear. This dimension of personality could be summarized as an aca-

demically oriented one in which the need to achieve is more likely to be realized than in the previous factor.

Factor VII: The abasive-dependent. Four variables are a part of this factor. One of these, the need, abasement, yields considerable influence, while the three values—succorance, nurturance, and the aesthetic values—have proportionately less. This factor is essentially self-effacing in nature, embodying needs to be taken care of and to care for others, and a sensitivity to beauty.*

The results indicate that the need pattern for nursing students is more complex than previous research has shown.

Clinical Studies

Another line of research concerned with unconscious as well as conscious motivating factors has utilized projective techniques to study the personality of the prototypical nursing student and to assess the factors that relate to success. The TAT (Thematic Apperception Test) has been used to take an in-depth look at the nursing student, tapping the role of conscious and unconscious motivation.

Cleveland (1961) administered four TAT cards and a questionnaire to 154 nursing students to investigate conscious and unconscious motivation for entering the profession. Unconscious factors revealed by the TAT involve a need to defend against feelings of suffering, discomfort, and anguish. When the study was repeated with graduate nurses, the results duplicated the entering student pattern but with greater intensity (that is, graduate nurses displayed a greater need for defences against impulses). The overall picture of the nursing student indicates that she is passive, nonachieving, melancholic, and had a depressive outlook on life and a tension-filled relationship with her parents.

The results of the questionnaire indicate that the primary conscious reason for entering nursing was the desire to serve mankind. The questionnaire also indicated that nursing students choose nursing as a career early in life. From this Cleveland reasoned that there are early and repressed personality dynamics involved in choosing nursing, and that the sort of person who would be most friendly and positive toward patients would be the one who empathizes with sickness and suffering. This personality would have tendencies to identify with sadness, misfortune, and role of the underdog.

Bernstein and others (1965) also attempted to assess the role of unconscious motivation in the choice of nursing as a career. They used all 20 TAT cards with a sample inventory of 67 nursing students, who were then compared with Eron's (1953) normative sample. Nursing students were more disturbed in their interpersonal relations than Eron's (1953) normative sample. Themes of need for succorance from parents and themes of physical harm inflicted or

*From Smith, J.E. 1968. Personality structure in beginning nursing students: A factor analytic study. *Nursing Research* 17:144.

wished upon parents by children were more apparent. There were a number of stories involving a child running away from home, the death or illness of a parent, or the illness of the child. Parental disappointment in the child, and the child's disappointment in the parents, were strong themes. Nursing students' test results exhibited more themes of separation and loneliness. Physical aggression, war, and fighting were strong themes. However, these themes were coupled with themes of retribution, such as legal restrictions and obligations to society. This suggests that impulses are strong but nursing students also have a strong defense structure.

Unlike Cleveland, Bernstein and others found strong achievement-oriented themes with few stories of inadequacies. A number of themes suggested sexual curiosity as an unconscious motivation for the selection of medicine as a career. Bernstein hypothesized that nursing is a safe and acceptable way to explore sexuality. He thought the themes indicated that the nursing students do not have satisfying, lasting relationships with people important to them (parents, boyfriends, girlfriends, etc.), but are normal in their peer group relations.

Bernstein and others view nursing as an occupational choice reflecting early parent-child experiences: "By entering nursing, relationships with patients are relatively short-term and superficial and yet serve the students' needs for approval." They suggest that the themes of greater hostility expressed by nurses in the TAT are ways for them to channel unacceptable impulses into a socially useful profession. Nursing procedures allow for the healing of patients and yet at the same time may hurt them. Bernstein and others explain the differences in achievement needs between their findings and Cleveland's findings as the result of using different TAT cards.

Edwards (1969) also compared nursing students with a normative population, this time a group of liberal arts majors. Edwards found the nursing students to be quiet, melancholic, conservatively dressed, with a childhood experience of illness, accident, or loss. Nursing students consistently preferred fantasy to reality and avoided intrapersonal and introspective depth. Themes of loneliness and a view of life as unpredictable, often futile, and controlled by fate were prominent. The nursing students tended to prefer fantasy boyfriends to actual relationships. There was a passive avoidance of sexuality and resignation to the loss of a love object. The nursing student saw herself as having a limited amount of femininity. The themes suggest that young women come from homes with an absence of the father-daughter interactions that reinforce a feminine image. The father was seen as either "strict," "conservative," or "reserved," and this was usually coupled with a dominant mother.

Edwards thought that individuals choose nursing because nursing meets some critical emotional needs. First, nursing is conducive to sexual fantasies in its demands. Nursing requires physical confrontation with patients that is both safe and sterile and provides confirmation of femininity within a structured and unthreatening situation. Libidinal energy is channeled into abstractions such as the "ministering angel." Edwards stressed that nursing education takes place when adolescent pressures are emerging, and maintains that nursing allows a safe defense against those rising pressures. (The woman's movement and the entrance of older married students into nursing may mean this is not as true of today's student as it was in 1969.)

Kibrick (1963), investigating the effect of self and role perception on dropouts from nursing school, also viewed the nursing student as defending herself against sexual and aggressive impulses. Students who remained in school were "nurturant" and "placed the welfare of others above their own personal interest." Continuing students were "submissive in their behavior" and "responsive to patients;" while students who withdrew "resented authority" and were "less willing to submit to the routines and practices of the school."

Although authors using the TAT have taken an in-depth look at the nursing student in their attempts to assess the complexity of the motivation, there appears to be little consideration of individual differences. Are all students entering nursing attempting to displace sexual and aggressive impulses? Although the data yielded by the TAT are in some ways more complex than those yielded by the EPPS or MMPI, the researchers assume there is one standardized personality pattern for all nursing students.

Results from studies using the TAT and the EPPS indicate that a number of personality needs are influential in the choice of nursing as a vocation. It appears that nursing is a safe way to express aggressive and sexual impulses and to have relationships involving the giving and taking of warm feelings. As such, it would most certainly appeal to the adolescent who needs a defense against the rising pressures of her sexuality. The findings, however, also indicate that no one personality represents the nursing student. The relationship is complex and there are several patterns that predict success in nursing education.

PERSONALITY PATTERNS OF SUCCESSFUL NURSING STUDENTS

My research (HEW, 1974) reveals three distinct personality types that are successful in nursing education.

In this study, the personality factors measured by the 16 P.F. and the attitudinal dimensions of the Image of Nursing Scale were analyzed using a nontraditional methodology (see Appendix C). Rather than constructing a single personality type of nursing student from these measures, a broader approach that could bring out different subsets within the sample was used.

The analysis was accomplished by collecting scores on the 16 P.F. and Image of Nursing Scale for 120 nursing students from four of the seven schools, dividing this group into two random subsamples, and subjecting each set of profiles to a cluster analysis by the method outlined by Howard and Gordan (1963). The general procedure involves identifying a cluster nucleus consisting of highly similar profiles and adding to these clusters other profiles similar to the cluster members. New clusters are started when no acceptable candidates can be found for inclusion in existing clusters. The procedure terminates when no new clusters can be identified.

Using this approach, preliminary results of the 16 P.F. and Image of Nursing Scale indicate that for each instrument, three different major (and several minor) typologies or clusters emerged. The 16 P.F. produced the following types:

Type One: This type can be designated as "modal." It did not differ on any of the scales from the standard sample used for comparison (college women in general). This group of students exemplifies Kardiner's (1945) "modal personality." The personality patterns reflect the prevailing cultural mores and psychological defenses.

Type Two: This type can be designated as "neurotic introvert." These individuals, as a group, are high on the anxiety and neurotic defense mechanism scales, and score low on the leadership scales. One subgroup within this general personality type scored highly in creativity, possibly indicating some outlet for the anxiety.

Type Three: This type can be characterized as "normal self-reliant." These individuals are low on the anxiety, neurosis, and leadership scales, and high on the scale measuring alert poise.

The Image of Nursing Scale questionnaire also produced three typologies; in this case, of attitudes toward the nursing profession.

Type One: The "modal" type holds an image of nursing similar to that held by society. The group mean for each dimension falls close to the overall mean for the reference group of nursing students.

Type Two: The "instrumental image." Individuals in this typology do not regard nursing either as having much importance in the social scheme, or as means to achieve personal satisfaction. Nursing is viewed, rather, as a means to future independence.

Type Three: The "expressive image." Individuals in this typology regard nursing as a good preparation for marriage, and a career that provides a great deal of personal satisfaction—in short, it is an avenue to a personally involving, good life. Their one complaint is the restriction of personal freedom during training.

These findings indicate that the single stereotypical nursing personality suggested in prior research does not exist, and that there is not a single stereotypical view of the nursing field. In this sample, three major personality typologies emerged, as well as specific profiles that did not fit into these categories. The same held true with the Image of Nursing typologies, where three distinct views of the field were found within this sample.

Relationships Between the Typologies

Analysis of the images of nursing (modal, instrumental, and expressive) and different personality typologies (modal, neurotic introvert, and normal self-reliant) reveal certain relationships. When three 16 P.F. personality typologies were correlated by the chi-square test with the types on the Image of Nursing questionnaire, two major relationships emerged: The neurotic introvert type (Type Two, 16 P.F.) was significantly correlated to the expressive image type (Type Three, Image). The modal personality type (Type One, 16 P.F.) was significantly correlated to the instrumental image type (Type Two, Image).

Most significantly, the expressive view of nursing (a nursing career is regarded as a road to the good life) was held by individuals who could be characterized as neurotic introverts (that is, they show a great deal of anxiety and a number of neurotic defense mechanisms). Apparently, young women with strong feelings of inadequacy and a depreciated self-concept are attracted to nursing because of the redemptive qualities they perceive in nursing. This substantiated my colleagues' and my impression of the students who took advantage of the counseling offered through a crisis intervention program—that is, a portion of the student body did indeed use nursing as a means to bolster their depreciated self-images. This left them vulnerable to many vicissitudes in the educational situation and more likely to go into crisis.

The instrumental view (nursing as a road to freedom) was held by individuals who fit into the modal personality typology. Apparently the normative young woman in pursuit of a nursing diploma does not value the field as highly as her fellow nursing students. This is not to say she has a negative view of the field, but she is not as enthused as the rest of her classmates. She is less concerned with the expressive aspects of nursing and the emotional satisfaction she will derive from her career than she is with the vocational freedom it will provide. Perhaps her emotional needs are being met in other ways, and she does not need nursing for emotional satisfaction.

An alternative explanation is that the instrumental view of nursing stems from problems in the professional socialization process. It is difficult to assume the nursing role and the corresponding responsibility, and one way to deal with the accompanying anxiety is to put emotional distance between oneself and the profession. The result is the instrumental view, in which a nursing student looks to the future for independence but not for personal satisfaction.

These relationships, however, do not exist in every school nor in the total sample. Data from each school were analyzed for school-specific typologies, which were tested for correlation with the demographic population and philosophy of education in the respective schools. It is apparent that different schools recruit different types of students as a function of the socioeconomic level within the school and the school's reputation in the community. As a result, different schools produced different percentages of each type of student.

RESULTS AND THEIR SIGNIFICANCE
FOR PROFESSIONAL SOCIALIZATION

What does this research indicate about the process of professional socialization? Does it support the contention that Stage II (resistance), a critical epi-
sode for professionalization, is not encouraged by the educational system?

Notwithstanding some confusion in the different instruments and meth-
odologies employed and in the results, certain findings emerge from the studies: Different personality patterns are common among nursing students, and
these patterns do correlate with completion of the program. Nursing students
as a group tend to be higher on deference, nurturance, and endurance, and
lower on dominance and autonomy than a comparison sample of college
women. There is an indication that parental relationships are built on tension,
and that these students are sad and likely to identify with the sick and the
underprivileged.

A comparison of dropouts and graduates showed that dropouts resemble
a standard college population in their need for achievement, deference, order,
endurance, and aggression (Reece, 1961). Kibrick (1963) found continuing students to be more nurturant and submissive in their behaviors and more responsive to patients.

The research presented in this chapter indicates that students who exhibit
Stage II resistance will have trouble graduating from a typical school of nursing. However, assuming they resemble a normal population in their adolescent
need for rebellion and questioning, nursing students must be unusually self-
reliant or able to conceal their aggression from the faculty, because a nursing
student who has trouble concealing anger or cannot sublimate rebellious needs
is in for trouble during her school years. She will most likely become one of the
students who make up Teal and Fabrizio's (1961) category of nonacademic
dropout.

RECENT DEVELOPMENTS

Most recent studies on nursing students have turned from studying the
causes of attrition in nursing education and attitudes and personality traits of
nurses toward examining the characteristics of applicants to nursing schools.
This shift in emphasis is due to the increasing numbers of students applying to
nursing schools (De Tornyay, 1977; Plummer and Phelan, 1976). As Willman
(1976) states: "One of the more signficant developments on the educational
scene in recent years is the fact that most nursing programs in the United States
are finding themselves in the enviable and unusual position of having many

more applicants than can be accommodated, despite the expansion of teaching facilities and faculties."*

There are several reasons for this. The expansion of the health care field accompanied by a declining educational system at the secondary level makes a nursing career lucrative in terms of finding a job after graduation. The increasing numbers of women working outside the home (partly a result of the women's liberation movement) and the movement to bring minorities into the mainstream means more people want to enter nursing. Finally, community colleges make nursing education available to individuals with limited funds. Willman points out that this results in the paradox of nursing attracting more qualified students as well as educationally disadvantaged students. Willman assumes that, with this heterogeneity, the educational structure will change to meet the diverse needs of the students and asserts that individualization is the key to this new structure. This individualization is to be accomplished through student-centered education, which respects and protects "the rights of the most able students along with the rights of disadvantaged students most in need of specialized help."

If this type of student-centered education takes place, the characteristics of nursing students would indeed change, and the research done in the 1960s would be interesting only as history. Is the system changing? Perhaps, but the recent literature on the traits of student nursing and graduates does not indicate this.

Ventura (1976), in examining traits such as dominance, responsibility, socialization, self-control, good impression, achievement via conformance, and achievement via independence in senior students enrolled in three different types of programs (B.S.N., diploma, and A.D.), found that B.S.N. students (who as "professional" students should show the most change) instead looked a great deal like the nursing students studied by Adams and Klein (1970). B.S.N. students were lower on dominance than A.D. students and were higher on self-control, good impression, and achievement via conformance than diploma students.

Rein (1977) found that although nursing students did not think they were dominant and that medical students wanted the nurses they met to be more dominant, nursing students portrayed their ideal nurse as very dominant. This is a good sign. However, the medical students did not want the ideal nurse to be as dominant as the nursing student wanted her to be.

Sullivan (1978) proposes that the old order has changed dramatically. In Sullivan's study, the EPPS revealed a significant shift from 1973 to 1978. The rank order of needs among nurses was strikingly different from that collected

*From Willman, M. Changes in nursing students. In *Current Perspectives in Nursing Education: The Changing Scene*, p. 74.

in previous samples. Need for heterosexuality, dominance, introception, change, and achievement consistently appeared highest since 1973, whereas need for deference, order, and endurance consistently scored among the lowest six needs. When Sullivan compared the nurses to a group of physicians, only one of the needs, introception, was found to differ significantly between the nurse and the physician groups, and the nurses scored higher. Sullivan concludes that "the shift in needs of the nurses and the high similarity of needs of the nurse and physician groups suggest an emerging assertiveness on the part of the nurses and a trend toward similarity of need patterns with physicians practicing in primary care."

Unfortunately, the sampling procedure and methodology utilized in this study leave Sullivan's results and conclusions open to question. The nursing sample was 129 graduate nurses enrolled in a short-term medical nurse-practitioner program between 1972 and 1976. These nurses were requested to take the EPPS during their first week of classes and 127 of the 129 complied. The corresponding physician sample was obtained from the physicians who had agreed to bring the nurses into practice with them, and they were mailed the test, with the request that they complete it in one sitting. Only 52% responded.[1] The differences in the responses of the physicians and nurses indicate that even a nurse-practitioner (viewed as the front line movement toward greater professionalism) has a long way to go before matching the physician's autonomy. Perhaps the nurses' reaction to the test is evidence of a habit of obedience and submission to authority. This could explain the incredibly high response rate and the results. Resentment is a natural reaction to a situation in which it appears that answering personal questions is mandatory.[2] This resentment could lead to dominance emerging as a high priority. The results of Sullivan's study are interesting but cannot be construed as evidence of a changing nursing personality.

NOTES

1. Several physicians who did not complete the schedule responded to explain why they did not: lack of time, lack of confidence in the confidentiality of the results, and the fact that the findings might be used inappropriately in the selection process were cited.
2. Sobol (1978) recognized the problems with voluntary versus mandatory participation in an article exploring B.S.N. students' self-actualization and response to stress. In the four schools studied, two offered class time and at these institutions participation ranged from 82% to 100%. In the third college, the instruments were taken out of class and only 52% of the students participated and in the fourth college the faculty reported that the students were unwilling to volunteer. Sobol thought that since nursing research is emphasized in all the colleges, the reluctance of the students in the third and fourth colleges should be of concern to the faculty. Sobol cites the Sheridan and Shack (1970) study which indicates that vol-

unteers are more self-accepting, less dependent, and more self-actualizing than nonvolunteers. This may be true in Sheridan and Shack's college population—however, among nursing students standing up for their rights has been extremely hazardous and nonparticipation might be a good sign.

Sobol's (1978) finding that self-sufficiency correlates with self-actualization (measured by Shostrom's Personal Orientation Inventory) is indeed significant. However, of equal, if not greater, significance is her recognition of the level of stress involved in nursing education. Initially she views this as a function of the rigorous program in theory and clinical practice, the discrepancy between the lay image of nursing and the reality of the process, the fear of making a potentially lethal error, and the skepticism of the other health professionals toward baccalaureate nursing education. After analyzing her results and realizing the variation between programs in respect to the students' anxiety levels and scores on the measure of self-actualization, she came to the conclusion that further study was needed in this area. The further study would include broadening the base of the sample of nursing students and studying the faculty and graduates who help socialize the student nurse. She recommends a more adult-centered approach to nursing education because it would produce greater self-direction and autonomy. Willman (1976) and Rosedahl (1974) agree. If these changes in the educational climate can indeed be implemented, the research done on nursing students in the 1980s will reflect a change in the "nursing personality." If only the form changes, the results will be the same as they were in the early 1970s and in the recent literature.

Chapter 7

A FEMALE PROFESSION

Florence Nightingale changed the role of women in nursing from camp follower to caretaker and nurturer. Prior to her time, only males had been allowed to nurse; it was assumed that any female who would take up this "base" profession would also be a prostitute. After Florence Nightingale, women were allowed into the profession, and in the years since, nursing has become an almost exclusively female occupation. (Even today, with more men entering the field, nursing is 97% female.[1])

Not only are the nurses' peers and supervisors likely to be female, but the general public expects nurses to demonstrate the female personality traits associated with nurturing and serving. In fact, so firmly entrenched are these traits in everyone's minds that the masculinity of any male nurse is questioned (Segal, 1962). The American public assumes that the male nurse must possess the traditional female traits of dependence, passivity, indecision, and inappropriate emotional reactions and involvements. How could he otherwise be a nurse?

Chapter 3 illustrated how latent identities, including sex and race, play a part in determining how easily a particular student or group of similar students passes through the stages of socialization. The greater the differences between the latent identity and the professional identity, the more predictable the students' role-identity problems would be—even in well-structured programs with ideally supportive cultural climates.

In our culture, nurses are expected to be maternal, caring, compassionate, and as emotionally involved with patients as mothers are with sick children (Schulman, 1958; Wilson, 1971). Physicians, on the other hand, can assume what Lief and Fox (1963) call "detached concern." The nurse is seen as the passive, unassertive, submissive, dependent female (Braverman and others, 1972); a foil to the decisive, aggressive, independent, dominant male father-figure physician. This gives rise to what Stein (1972) calls the doctor-nurse game, where the nurse pursues professional ends by manipulation—flirting and suggesting—rather than in a straightforward manner. Bullough (1975), in "Barriers to the Nurse-Practitioner Movement: Problems of

Women in a Woman's Field,'' views these cultural expectations as the predominant barrier to the nurse-practitioner movement:

> It has been shown that the doctor-nurse game and the anticipatory withdrawal of nurses at both the microcosmic and macrocosmic levels have created formidable barriers to the nurse-practitioner movement. Viewed from the historical and sociological perspectives, the difficulties which nurse-practitioners have faced in gaining acceptance are easier to understand. The sex segregation in medicine and nursing and the subordinate role of women in the past helped establish traditions, which, when nurtured in the exploitive atmosphere of the hospital training schools, created patterns of interaction between nurses and physicians [that are] obstacles to the full use of talents of both professions.*

Since the early sixties many studies have found that these traditional female traits interfere with the nurse's professional orientation. Meyer (1960) categorizes nurses into four types, based on their views of what was most valuable about nursing care. At one end of the continuum are Type I nurses, who place the highest value on patient care and resemble the mother surrogate image of the nurse; at the other extreme are Type IV nurses, who value the technical administration tradition and emphasize planning and supervision of functions to be carried out by other workers. Meyer characterizes Types II and III as different versions of the modern nurse. Both these types prefer work situations in which the nurse shares her patients with colleagues. The modern nurse resolves the diverse appeals of Types I and IV by choosing to work with both patients and colleagues. What differentiates Type II from Type III is a preference for either patients or colleagues. Type II places the colleague relationships first. Type III, although wishing to work with both staff and patients, places patient relationships first.

Senior nursing students seem oriented toward the technical-professional values of Type IV. In Meyer's longitudinal study, freshman students valued Type I (ministering angel) most, whereas Type II (modern nurse) was valued by seniors. This change in values is most striking for B.S.N. students but is also true of diploma school students. A.D. students do not show the same changes as the other two groups. Meyer concludes:

> While it is not within the province of the researcher to evaluate these changes, it does seem that the regular increase of Type II approximates the goals of nursing today. The philosophy of team nursing as outlined by Lambertsen and Newcomb (1953) stresses the sharing process and depends on the capacity of the professional nurse to value her teammates and at the same time the team. Type II nurses seem most likely to fulfill this role.**

Wilson (1971) also calls for a movement away from the mother surrogate

---

*From Bullough, B. 1975(a). Barriers to the nurse practitioner movement: Problems of women in a women's field. *International Journal of Health Services* 5(2):309-317.
**From Meyer, G.R. 1960. *Tenderness and Technique: Nursing Values in Transition.* Calif.: Institute for Industrial Relations.

image of nursing: "Nurses . . . must develop a sense of self-identity, independent and different from the culturally ascribed roles." The old virtues of intuition, nurturance, and dependency must be replaced by those of intellect, productivity, and independence, she argues. Lewis (1976) and Santo (1978) are upset because the work situation for the newly graduated nurse and the internship experience for a nurse-practitioner still do not foster intellectual curiosity, productivity, or independence.

Schulman (1972) rejects his earlier analysis of the nursing role as primarily maternal. He speculates that the specialization of physicians (which created an increased need for competent, specialized assistants) and internal changes in the nursing field (which pressed for increasing professionalism and control over the job situation) changed the nursing role from one of emotional attachment toward the patient to the detached concern of the medical profession.

Schmidt (1968), when considering the evolution of the field, recognizes the dichotomy between the mother surrogate/ministering angel and the professional nurse. Schmidt concludes by addressing this problem:

> Nursing cannot turn back to the traditional images of the ministering angel if this means becoming any less professional and technically competent. The way forward for nursing tends also towards the "human side" of patient care. Thus the ideal image of the nurse for the future would appear to call for a special blending of the old Nightingale spirit with the new, which calls for professional skills. Perhaps the lamp as a symbol of nursing can still serve its purpose—providing nurses come to combine with the light of the lamp (professional skills) the warmth of the light (supportive personal response).*

Traditional female traits, as exemplified in Meyer's Type I nurse, are the antithesis of professionalism that expresses detached concern. Indeed, many researchers appear to define professionalism along the lines of the currently prevalent model of professionalism—the male. If nurses exemplify traditional female traits and if male traits define the professional role, then Schmidt's proposal to integrate the two is a monumental task.

It is appropriate to examine the effect of this contradiction on the education of the nursing student. Three factors will be examined: first, students' motivations for choosing nursing as a career, which illuminate the link between the student's female identity and her image of the nursing role; second, sex-role ideologies and entering nursing students' particular interpretation of femininity; and third, a student's progression through the four stages of socialization, which should culminate in the resolution of the conflict between the feminine and professional roles. The final section in this chapter contains an analysis of the effect of sex-role stereotyping on professionalism in nursing and proposed solutions.

*From Schmidt, M.H. 1968. Role conflict. *American Journal of Nursing* 68:2348-2350.

The Choice of Nursing as a Career

Traditionally, students enter nursing for nurturant reasons: they want to help people. In my study of 734 entering diploma students, two-thirds of the sample chose nursing because they thought taking care of people was important. Additionally, 80% of the sample agreed with the statement: "More than any other occupation for women, nursing provides opportunities for worthwhile services to humanity." This substantiates Meyer's (1960) earlier finding that the majority of entering students in all three types of educational programs hold Type I (ministering angel) images of nursing. Other researchers have reported similar findings (Simpson and Simpson, 1969; Katz and Martin, 1972; Schoenmaker and Radosevich, 1976).

The caretaking motivation is viewed by most researchers as a component of the female personality, in opposition to other career-choice motivations such as scientific interest, job security, and advancement possibilities, which are considered to be masculine components. Further, Katz and Martin (1972) hypothesize that students not only choose nursing for traditionally feminine reasons, but they do so in a typically feminine manner. Katz and Martin (1972) found, and my research confirms, that many nursing students are uncertain as to when or why they chose nursing. A frequent response to the question, "Why did you choose nursing?" was "I don't know; I have always wanted to be a nurse." The vagueness of this answer, compared to the more explicit reasons presented by males who chose medicine, are characteristic of female career choice patterns (Katz and Martin, 1972).

Nurses choose nursing as a career almost as early as physicians choose medicine, a decision found to be one of the earliest career decisions (Rogoff, 1957; Barnartt, 1976). Unlike medicine, nursing is chosen without rational considerations of alternatives, and without eliminating other possible careers. This early choice, combined with the vague rationale, suggests that the choice is linked to the female role and helps provide her with an identity at adolescence. As such, it becomes a cornerstone of the young woman's identity around which other aspects of her identity will be built (Erikson, 1950). Whatever view of the nursing role educators or practitioners may have, the student enters convinced that nursing is nurturant and feminine at its core, and this may well be her reason for choosing nursing.

Sex-Role Identities in Entering Nursing Students

Nursing students enter school with humanitarian values. They score higher on humanitarian scales than beginning medical students (Eron, 1955; Moody, 1973). They are idealistic, and this idealism is related to their female interpretation of the nursing role. They emphasize those virtues considered female in our society and transfer them into necessary professional traits. For example, Psathas (1969) found that freshmen tended to emphasize the emotional support rather than the technical side of nursing. Upon entrance, these students also score high on scales of femininity. Levitt and other (1962) found that B.S.N. students had significantly lower scores on such masculine scales as autonomy, aggression, and dominance than did a comparison group of female college students. Similar personality traits have been found by other researchers (Redden and Scales, 1961; Bailey and Claus, 1969; Edwards, 1969).

Nursing is picked for traditionally female reasons, and students expect nursing to be secondary to their main interest in life — families-to-be. In my study of diploma nurses, 90% of the sample expected their families to come first, and most of them planned a combined career as nurse, wife, and mother. Sixty percent of the students thought studying nursing could prepare them for family life. Davis and Olesen (1965) found similar results among baccalaureate students. In their study, 87% of the students expected their families to come first. Furthermore, their longitudinal data show that this ranking did not change over time as students progressed toward graduation.

Changes in Sex-Role Identity
During the Educational Years

Interestingly, these humanitarian attitudes are stable over time despite onslaught from the educators. Schools of nursing typically try to inculcate attitudes that reflect the primary values of knowledge of the field and technical competence. There is no doubt that nursing faculties prefer the Type IV nurse (professional) to the Type I nurse (ministering angel).

How do students react to these attempts to change their attitudes? Meyer (1960) did find a diminution in the number of students holding the Type I image. However, she also found differences by type of program (a topic that has not been investigated fully and deserves more attention). Davis and Olesen (1964) found that the change toward a more detached professional view did take place, but the number of students who changed was small. The entire class approved of the idea that demonstrating care and concern were the primary values in nursing; after one year only 10% had changed their minds. Furthermore, Olesen and Whittaker (1968), in analyzing the same students and how they had changed throughout their 4 years in school, found that these students explicitly objected to the lack of femininity in the faculty's view of their future career role. They expressed their resistance in open objections, in grieving and mourning for their former, more comfortable roles, and in conning their instructors so that they looked professional in conversations with the instructors even if they did not believe what they were saying.

Some changes in the humanitarian values and idealism are evident in the course of the educational process. Seniors show more technical and less idealistic values than freshmen (Psathas, 1969). Other studies indicate that scores in humanitarianism are slightly lower for advanced students than for freshmen. However, this small change in attitudes and values attests to the strength of the motivation that brings women into nursing and to the importance of the nurturant view of nursing in their self-concepts.

How Sex Roles Affect
the Stages of Socialization

Students choose nursing as a profession because they have a desire to nurture, and the prototypical entering student holds a traditional view of the female sex role. She also expects nursing to enhance her ability to play this role. Since the students enter with high scores on scales measuring dependency, compliance, and submissiveness, students should have no trouble with Stage I, which requires dependence, compliance, and trust. However, although they are predisposed to comply with the image of the professional nurse fostered by faculty and administration, this image collides with their view of femininity. The resulting clash leads to Stage II, negative/independence, as postulated by our model.

Olesen and Whittaker's (1968) study on B.S.N. students details how students cope with the conflict inherent in their desire to be nurturing and female and the faculty's demands for objective, scientific, and what students perceive as masculine behavior. They grieve and mourn for their old, more comfortable, feminine roles, and they con their instructors with the appearance of agreeing with faculty values while retaining their old values. Paradoxically, the demands of nursing education for a switch to a more professional, technical, and objective view of the field propels the students into a mode of behavior that the faculty finds difficult to tolerate — resistance. It is no wonder that Olesen and Davis (1966) found that construction of the student's role image was quite complicated.

These students did not wish to give up their image of the nurse as a ministering angel, but attempted to add professional and leadership qualities to that image, despite inherent inconsistencies. Understandably, the change in values and attitudes demonstrated by the students varies considerably. Some students completely give up their image of nursing as a female nurturant occupation, while others steadfastly maintain this image in the face of strong opposition.

These problems in Stages I and II set the stage for transition to mutuality, Stage III, in which students should use the peer group as a testing ground for various ways of playing the nursing role. According to Olesen and Davis' study, Stage III does exist. Students do test out the faculty's admonitions on behavior together and try to find a way to utilize their previous identities in playing the new role. The fact that the students in Olesen and Davis' sample (1966) did not give up their view of the nurse as ministering angel but tried to combine it with the image promulgated by the faculty indicates that they are struggling with the tasks of Stage III. They are trying to incorporate the professional role into previous roles and resolve the discrepancy between their latent identities and the role demands of the professional. When they reach Stage IV (interdependence), students should be able to integrate their professional and personal selves.

Meyer's data (1960) indicates that the amount of change in the image of the field varies from program to program; thus the successful resolution of Stage III depends on the idiosyncratic characteristics of schools or perhaps on the classes within schools. This is dangerous for the nursing profession, since it means that resolution of this important stage is not structured into the system but left to chance.

The resolution of Stages II and III is dependent upon the psychological and sociological variables previously discussed. These variables tend to be considered in the abstract by nurse educators without extensive research into how the reality of nursing is matching the concepts. Furthermore, there is a lack of integration of the sociological and psychological variables so that researchers in one area do not consider the other.

This integration depends on successful resolution of the conflict in Stage II. The next section examines how the traditional female role conflicts with the professional role, observes how nursing students react to this incongruence, and suggests ways to remedy this situation.

FEMALE NURSES AND
THE PROFESSIONAL ROLE

Researchers and society in general tend to label dominance, autonomy, and professionalism as masculine traits, leading to the conclusion that females with more masculine attitudes can best adapt to the professional role of nurse. Stromberg (1976) found that those nursing students with more "masculine" self-images held more professional images of the nursing role. Tetreault (1976) concurred, and asserted that students with more professional attitudes toward nursing hold a more active (and hence more masculine) role identity than students with less professional attitudes did.

This confusion between masculinity and autonomy leaves the nursing student between Scylla and Charybdis. If she becomes professional, she loses her femininity; if she retains her femininity, she loses professional acceptance. This paradox sets the climate for the resistance of Stage II. Nursing students' feminine motivations and sex role ideologies have been part of their personalities since birth and are the cornerstone of their identities.

The professional image of nursing should not and does not rule out the nurturant aspects of patient care. Nursing students are not taught to reject this image; however, few emerge with the conceptual tools to integrate nurturance with the technical and professional aspects of nursing. Perhaps this is because nursing researchers and educators have fallen into the trap of defining professionalism in the framework of *male* professionalism.

Why does this happen? Probably because nursing lacks a clear-cut theoretical base to define the nursing role and functions and set priorities; and because there is a dearth of role models for neophytes to follow.

Simpson and Simpson (1969) discuss the problems that arise in what they term a semiprofession.[2] Lacking a firm theoretical base, the specific tasks in a semiprofession are ill-defined. A variety of tasks are possible, ranging from technical and specific to emotional and general. This vagueness about the relative importance of various aspects of the field makes it easy for one aspect such as emotional care to be emphasized by some, and another aspect such as knowledge and technical competence to be emphasized by others. This leads to confusion for teachers, practitioners, and students. In nursing the problem is compounded because nurses work with physicians (classified by Simpson and Simpson as a true profession). Knowledge and technical competence are the base of the physician role. This becomes the definition of "professional" in the health care field. With the tradition of male physicians and female nurses, masculine comes to mean professional. Those wishing to upgrade nursing to a true profession on par with the physician stress the masculine qualities needed in nursing. The traditional structure of the health care field makes it difficult to assert that many of the values described as feminine and therefore nonprofessional are human values and can be part of a professional role.

This confusion between femininity and professionalism is perpetuated by the lack of role models who successfully portray an autonomous and professional interpretation of the role. The role models (those faculty members in contact with the students) have probably done little to resolve for themselves the conflict between a masculine, aggressive professionalism promulgated by those who wish to upgrade the profession, and their own idealistic desire to be feminine and nurturant. Indeed, many of them left nursing practice for teaching to escape this conflict.

Where does this leave the newly graduated nurse? Perhaps part of Kramer's (1974) reality shock is reconciling the female role expectations and the professional role. Ideally, the new graduate should approach her career as a professional, secure because she has a body of knowledge and skills that merit professional recognition. With this as armor, she could cope with the work situation and fight for changes in those practices detrimental to her profession, her patients, and the institution in which she works. Her goals and self-concept will be well-defined, and she should see no contradiction between statements such as "I want to help people" or "My family comes first" and the professionalism demanded by the nursing profession. These statements reflect, after all, human values, and professionalism should not preclude humanitarianism.

There is no reason why nurturance, in specific scientific and objectively designated ways, could not be part of the conceptualization of the nursing role. The definition of professionalism must be expanded to include more than the physician's role and its corresponding characteristics. To this end, a definitive theoretical base for professional nursing operations must be decided upon. Specific tasks performed solely by nurses must be developed, and these tasks must stem directly from a theory that will assign priorities to the tasks. If nursing moves toward this specific conceptualization of its place in the health care professions, the present dichotomy between masculine professionalism, and the femaleness of nursing, can disappear.

At present, nursing is questioning the motivations that prompt individuals to choose the field. This conflict is difficult for both students and practitioners. Perhaps less attention should be directed toward the type of educational program necessary to produce the professional nurse, and more attention paid to conceptualizing the role. This type of conceptualization could begin by resolving the current conflict between culturally defined femininity and "masculine" professionalism.

NOTES

1. *American Nurses' Association Sample Survey of Registered Nurses.* 1977. Bureau of Health Manpower Division of Nursing, U.S. Public Health Service. Department of Health, Education, and Welfare.
2. Teaching, social work, and librarianship are also classified as semiprofessions. A more extensive discussion of nursing and its theoretical base is in Chapter 10.

Chapter 8

MINORITY STUDENTS
IN NURSING

What happens when students not typical of those already in the field enter a profession? How do they integrate their previous roles with the expectations of the socializers? What is the educational experience like when the students do not share the faculty's covert norms and values? Do these students emerge with the internalized values prevalent in the field and the professional identities similar to the socializers' identities? Do they emerge at all, or do they simply drop out before graduation?

There is a dearth of literature on the problems minority students encounter in the socialization process. Most studies focus on the educational structure and suggest ways to remedy gaps in the students' educational background. The literature emphasizes remediation because "minority student" usually implies black and high-risk, or educationally disadvantaged. Clearly, this confuses the issue. Before the affirmative action programs, many black students had entered nursing. However, at that time there was no reason to consider them apart from the main group of students being educated and being socialized into the profession. Affirmative action programs caused schools to begin recruiting black students in greater numbers—not just black students but underprivileged, educationally disadvantaged, black students. Since these students had educational deficiencies that would almost certainly prevent them from graduating, the primary focus of programs and investigators necessarily was to remediate deficiencies and assure graduation.

This chapter analyzes the professional socialization process of a group of black high-risk students recruited into a diploma school of nursing.

BACKGROUND: HOW THIS GROUP
ENTERED A SCHOOL OF NURSING

The 32 high-risk minority students from which the data was drawn was a sample constituted by accident. They became an unplanned part of an HEW demonstration project designed to prevent attrition of nonrisk, prototypical (read "middle-class white") nursing students.

The HEW project, which was based on psychological intervention for emotional problems, had been designed to offer two types of support services: Crisis intervention consisting of individual counseling for specific emotional problems for up to eight 1-hour sessions; and motivational groups in which students with academic problems could gain an understanding of the emotional basis for their underachievement.

These services were augmented by a third support service, remedial tutoring in math and reading, because the director of the school had over the previous decade noted growing inadequacies in secondary school preparation. When the HEW grant application was made, the program was not designed to provide service for the educationally disadvantaged.

The rationale for the program was based on findings by Teal and Fabrizio (1961) and on the school director's observation of her students, both of which indicated that emotional rather than academic problems were the major cause of attrition. When the grant was received, the target class of 1970 had already been recruited, and was in no way different from the classes that had preceded them.

However, prior to the entrance of the target class, a new administration took over the direction of the school, changing the organizational structure and (at least implicitly) its philosophy of education. (See Appendix B for a summary of the HEW Grant findings.) More important was the fact that the new administration brought about a drastic change in the composition of the target class.

A special summer program had been sponsored by the school, aimed at recruiting students from the lower-income, inner-city black and Latino communities. The program consisted of remedial reading, writing, and mathematics and was designed to improve the students' basic skills to the school entrance requirements. At the end of summer, an administrative decision was made to admit 32 of the 45 summer students on the basis of their improvement in math and reading. Their NLN scores, which would have made their admission into a regular nursing program unthinkable, were disregarded. Predictive failure rate of the 32 was 100%. However, since the 32 high-risk minority students became part of the 1970 target class, they accordingly were served by the program.

The major thrust of the program for all students was the use of motivational group techniques, developed by Roth (1970). Usually the failing but academically competent student is assumed to lack the motivation to succeed. Roth's previous research had indicated that the underachiever (that is, a failing student whose academic predictors had indicated success) is indeed motivated, but motivated to fail. Underachievement is a way of life, and rather than renounce this and enter into a mature existence, the student prefers failure. As a result, the true underachievers are not candidates for voluntary counseling programs.

Roth proposed a confrontation type of group therapy experience for the underachiever, which would be mandatory for all failing students. In the presence of peers and a leader, the individual confronts her own will to fail. The group process prevents the rationalization formerly used to explain and justify failure. Developing relationships with group members facilitates acceptance of these insights without depression, and the individual can use the group experience to free herself from fear of and dependence upon authority figures.

In the HEW Grant program, the motivational groups were supplemented by both the crisis program (used for students diagnosed as inappropriate for the motivational groups and as a subsidiary resource to deal with problems that could not be resolved in the 15 weeks and by the remediation program (used to remedy deficiencies in basic skills).

Much to the surprise of everyone (including the director of the project), the treatment approach designed for one characterological problem (the underachiever with academic potential) worked remarkably well with motivated but academically deprived inner-city high-risk students. Table 8-1 shows the success rates for the different types of students and the various treatments.

A hypothesis is that motivational groups utilizing Roth's confrontation techniques make these inner-city students see themselves as architects of their own fate — a realization that comes as quite a shock to some students. The students were instructed to look to themselves rather than to others for causes and solutions. The motivational group leaders tried to convince the students that, while undoubtedly there was some cause for complaint about their environment and about the school, in some instances crying racism was a defense mechanism for rationalizing failure. This approach broke up the students' initial resistance to the remediation program, which they considered an insult to their intelligence and abilities. When the students began to use rather than avoid academic remediation and to view themselves as individuals who were behind but capable of catching up, the probability of their success was increased.

Intervention techniques used with this inner-city population, could no longer be fitted into the simple 15-week, 2-hour-per-week sessions without subsidiary services. Other programs offered by the project aided these students throughout their academic career. A black counselor and young graduate nurses, called "Gatekeepers," were assigned to mingle with the students,

TABLE 8–1   Treatment vs. Nontreatment Success/Failure Rates by Type of
             Admission Category (n = 98)*

	Regular Students	Regular Risk Students	Summer Risk Students
1. Treatment sample (n = 54)			
Group treatment †			
Success (n = 22)	11	5	6
Failure (n = 13)	6	4	3
Individual treatment			
Success (n = 17)	11	1	5
Failure (n = 3)	2	1	0
Total treatment			
Success (n = 39)	22	6	11
Failure (n = 16)	8	5	3
2. Nontreatment sample (n = 44)			
Refusing treatment			
Success (n = 5)	4	0	1
Failure (n = 21)	4	3	14
Never in need of treatment			
Success (n = 8)	8	0	0
Failure (n = 0)	0	0	0
Total nontreatment			
Success (n = 13)	12	0	1
Failure (n = 21)	4	3	14
3. Nonacademic withdrawals (n = 10)‡	5	2	3

*Other reports show 89 students because the records department did not list as part of the
class the 9 students withdrawing during orientation week.
†Students receiving both group and individual treatment are included only in group
treatment data.
‡These students withdrew before midterms, so no grades available. All were in extreme
psychological stress states and referred for treatment elsewhere.

coach them to play the nursing role appropriately, and discover the students'
problems. Care was taken by the gatekeepers so that students would not feel
that they were being spied on by the professional staff.

The crisis counselors and tutors were continually involved with the
minority students. Moreover, the faculty frequently took a hand and insisted
that the students utilize the remediation services, particularly when the students had no inclination to do so. As a result my staff and I knew these students far better than we knew the prototypical white students in the program at
the same time.

One constant comment from the staff during the three years of these students' education was, "These students certainly are different." The students were angrier, more sophisticated, and in many ways more realistic about the profession than were the nonminority students. The minority students were in the same age range as the rest of the students (19 to 22 years), but they were considerably farther along life's developmental path. Many were married, some had children, and some were married and divorced. Their latent identities and previously assumed roles were different from the white middle-class students who entered at the same time. The differences in latent identities were derived from the discrepancy between the social class groups. The students, however, thought it was their race that set them apart. They developed a group spirit based upon being black, which resulted in a powerful Black Students' Association. The white students had no organization that could match this; the student council was fragmented and disorganized.

The black students' school spirit contrasted dramatically with the behavior of the prototypical nursing student. Among the white students there was a lack of school spirit and interest in organizing that was typical for the school, which traditionally had an apathetic student body. However, the faculty did not always appreciate the demonstrations of black school spirit. The students, led by blacks, insisted upon, and finally received, an end to most dormitory rules, including supervision of hours, prohibition of males in the dormitory, and maid inspection of their rooms. Martin Luther King's birthday became a celebrated holiday. While many faculty members, in the abstract, appreciated the demands made by these students, there was continual fury over the rude manner in which the demands were presented. Interestingly, students in prior years had made many of these demands in a manner approved by the faculty and administration, but had never achieved their aims.

ANALYSIS OF THE SOCIALIZATION STAGES FOR THE MINORITY STUDENTS

In which stage of the socialization model were the black students when they entered nursing school? Where did they stand in the three spheres, and where were they developmentally when they finally acquired their diplomas?

Immediately apparent to everyone was that trust was to be a serious issue, since the latent identities of the faculty and the students did not match. This was a two-way street; the faculty no more trusted the students than the students trusted the faculty, and from the beginning, a cold war existed between the two groups, with occasional hot battles.

An example of the type of skirmish that broke out continually was the cry of racism by a well-endowed black student who was sent off the ward by her instructor for not wearing a bra. She stated (accurately) that the white students in her group were similarly braless, and contended that she was the object of overt discrimination. What became apparent to the black counselor who investigated the incident was that changing cultural norms, and basic physiognomy, rather than racism, caused the incident. The instructor, although young, had not realized that norms governing apparel had changed, and that few students wore bras under their heavily starched uniforms. With most of the white students it did not matter because they were not so well-endowed and the absence of a bra could not be detected. This black student's bralessnesss was more conspicuous.

What about similarly well-endowed white students? Here the difference between the two groups in the compliance of the first stage becomes apparent. The white, middle-class, well-endowed students knew they would be reprimanded if they went braless and, therefore, conformed to the expectations. They had no desire to become conspicuous over what they considered a trifle. In contrast, the black student viewed the instructor's interest in her undergarments as an infringement on her autonomy.

The black students were not as idealistic about nursing as the prototypical nursing students of previous years and Psathas' (1968) entering nursing students. They did not have what is termed an "expressive" view of nursing. They did not view nursing as the royal road to a good life in which they could become better wives and mothers by being nurses, or put their religious beliefs into effect and serve humanity. The lack of this attitude was revealed on the Image of Nursing Questionnaire, and constantly demonstrated in counseling sessions and in conversations with the faculty. It was especially apparent in the freshman *Orientation to Nursing* course and in the senior *History of Nursing* course.

The minority students were pragmatic; they took an "instrumental" view of nursing. Nursing was considered a route to freedom: a good job with a good salary. The faculty expected a more idealistic view of the field.

Since trust was limited if not nonexistent on both sides, these students did not readily accept the content of courses. They were continually questioning the purpose of learning the material presented and its relevance to a working nurse, the importance of professional issues and the value of knowing about insurance now (when, after all, they were not yet in the field).

Analyzing this behavior in terms of our model, it was hypothesized that these black students entered nursing school in Stage II. They arrived convinced that they would be treated differently because they were black, and since they had serious problems with basic skills, the faculty did indeed look askance at admitting this group. The students questioned faculty intentions and the material being presented. They began doubting whether the faculty members were as good at their job as they claimed to be and whether they really knew the material as they professed to know it. The students quickly banded together for group support which encouraged Stage II types of resistance by reinforcing the attitude that the students were right and the faculty was wrong.

The black counselor and the gatekeepers attached to the HEW project facilitated these students' moving into Stage III, mutuality. Students could try on the new professional role with people they trusted and respected, and could try to integrate their previous values and role behavior with the professional values and role behavior promulgated by the socializers. The success of Stage III and the help of the gatekeepers who served as role models and provided guidance made possible an occasional cease-fire, which permitted learning to take place.

It became apparent in the students' senior year that those who were indeed going to graduate were those who had taken advantage of the remedial programs and the psychological help available to them. Further, these students were progressing in a way that the prototypical white students who had not received this support and help were not. The students whose academic predictor scores prognosticated 100% chance of failure were the students who, as new graduates, most easily assumed the manner of the professional, integrated themselves into the hospital structure, and were quickly promoted to positions of power.

This group also reported greater satisfaction with hospital working conditions and, most importantly, with nursing and the nursing profession. There is no evidence whatsoever that they experienced reality shock. They had learned the hospital system well as nursing students and were for the most part contented, full-fledged professionals. The success of this group of students substantiates the contention that attachment to the field depends upon experiencing Stage II (resistance) and Stage III (mutuality).

The black students entered with latent identities so dramatically different from those of the faculty that the first stage of trust was completely disrupted. Stage II resistance began immediately. Without the demonstration project and the consistent efforts by the psychologists, the black counselor, and the gatekeepers to help the students overcome their academic handicaps and their emotional problems, the students almost certainly would have failed. However, these students graduated better socialized into the professional role than the more prototypical students, whose latent identities matched those of the socializers. The white students had neither academic nor emotional problems to hinder their progress through the socialization stages, but nevertheless were unprepared for the professional role at graduation. If this sample is typical of minority high-risk students, the lack of fit between their latent identities and the socializers' identities is not necessarily bad.

This type of student will probably be more resistive to the faculty than the prototypical student, and her progress will depend upon how the faculty handles this resistance. If it is suppressed and the problems are considered to be the student's, the student does not have a chance. If, however, the student receives help in closing the gap between the norms and values and those of the professionals directing the educational process, the student will emerge well-socialized into the profession.

Chapter 9

CASE STUDIES: PORTRAITS OF SUCCESS AND FAILURE

All happy families resemble each other; each unhappy family is unhappy in its own way.   Leo Tolstoy

When I began HEW project (1974), I assumed that all successful (that is, graduating) students would resemble each other, but the dropouts would fail in distinct and separate ways. This was a misconception. In both categories there were different roads to the goal. Several distinct patterns of intellectual, personality, and demographic factors emerged for both the successful and unsuccessful student.[1]

Francine: A Success Story

Successful in school and at ease with herself, Francine is a very intelligent young woman of 22. If a producer were looking for a prototypical nursing student to cast as "Cherry Ames, 1974," Francine would land the part. She is pretty, bright, well-liked by the faculty, and admired by her fellow students. A closer look reveals a person who would be better cast as the producer than a sweet and submissive student. Her personality dynamics do not resemble the personality patterns found in the nursing literature. She is not depressed or submissive, nor does she use nursing to defend against her sexual or aggressive impulses. She is self-possessed, confident, and sure of her ability to persuade others. She is not constrained by the stereotypic female role. Her future goal is to reorganize the health care field and the place of nursing with that field.

On our factors of the 16 P.F., she emerges as the prototype of the normal self-reliant student. She is low on the anxiety, neurosis, and leadership scales, and high on the scale measuring alert poise. She combines the instrumental and expressive image of nursing. She views nursing as a means to future independence and as a career offering a great deal of personal satisfaction. That is, she believes it will be satisfying once she restructures the field.

Francine could have gone to medical school but elected instead to become a nurse. How did this come about? Both of her parents are involved in health care delivery. Her father is a physician; her mother was an x-ray technician before she married. Francine had three years of college work in the biological sciences and applied to medical school. She was put on a waiting list and advised to complete her undergraduate work. Instead, while waiting for the next year and a place in the entering class, she took time off from school and worked in a hospital management position. During this year she observed the work and life styles of both physicians and nurses. When she received her admittance papers from the medical school, she declined and enrolled in a school of nursing instead.

Her reason for choosing nursing over the more prestigious role of physician was not based on the hard work or the long hours but on the type of relationship each has with the patient. She is convinced that the medical profession is making a mistake by allowing physicians to become specialized, less involved with the patients, and removed from their psychological needs. She thinks that the health care field must turn toward a preventive rather than a disease-oriented philosophy, and that when it does the nurse will be the prime agent in this type of treatment. She believes nurses should assess the needs of the patient, prescribe the regimes necessary to maintain health, or restore it as the case may be, physicians should be called in case of technical difficulty when specialized expertise is necessary.

Francine is also unusual in her conception of the place of nursing in her life. Most students plan to stay home with their children and resume their careers after the youngest is in school full time. They do expect to combine nursing with being wives and mothers but will give the family top priority. Francine, however, is sure she can combine the three and sees no reason to take time out for having a family. In *Passages*, Gail Sheehy (1974) describes some women as integrators, who manage to combine family, parenting, and career. Generally these women have either postponed their career or their nurturing until their thirties. Sheehy doubts that anyone in their early twenties can cope with juggling the demands of the three roles. Francine does not doubt her ability to do this and intends to start right after graduation.

Her profile on our psychological tests indicates that she should be able to integrate the demands of a family and a career. The second-order scores on the 16 P.F. provide a convenient capsule description of personality. Francine scored high on "tough poise," which indicates an enterprising, decisive, imperturbable personality. She also scored high on "independence," a sign of an aggressive, independent, self-directing personality. The Identity Scale indicates that she is comfortable with her career choice and has a positive evaluation of herself. She is high in "integrity" and "autonomy within social limits."

The Sentence Completion test reveals a well-integrated woman who had experienced some sibling rivalry. She feels close to her family but not dependent upon them. To the stem, "When they try to get me to be like my mother," she replies, "They wouldn't dare try." To the stem, "When they try to get me to be like my father," she replies, "I am already like him. We are both professionals." She thinks she has surpassed her brother (a medical student) because she feels he is blindly following the family tradition. She, on the other hand, has evaluated the family goals and chosen a path for herself. She believes her decision to become a nurse indicates that she has more sensitivity and autonomy than her brother and will be more successful.

She has problems in interpersonal relationships because she tends to pull away if the relationship becomes more than a superficial one. On the 16 P.F. she shows up high on the aloofness scale. Her TAT reveals a fear of intimacy and a preference to hold others at a distance. Her classmates' opinion of her reflects this problem. She is admired and regarded as a good spokesperson for the group, but she is not well liked. One of her classmates stated, "I like studying with her, I always vote for her when she wants to run any project, and she can be my spokesperson any time she wants. But I'd hate to room with her and I don't really like her very much. She makes me uncomfortable." Francine is aware of her classmates' opinions. She is aloof and judgmental. She does not want to become involved with most of her classmates except on a superficial basis. She is contemptuous of many of the other students and of the faculty. She wonders how they dared enter the field and why they feel they have the right to go forth and tend sick people when they lack judgment and knowledge. She has no tolerance for mistakes — others' or her own. She claims that a good professional never makes mistakes and that the good of the patient is always paramount. In this she resembles the "super nurse" ideal of many nurses. However, she is as critical of physicians as she is of herself and other nurses.

How did these personality dynamics affect her progress through the stages of socialization? It appears she was in Stage IV when she entered nursing school. Her early mentors were her parents, and she trusted their portrayal of health care professionals as good people involved in important work. Her rebellion against the system was apparently worked through during the year she took off and observed nurses and physicians in action. She does not use her peer group to practice trying on the professional role because she plans to restructure this role in the future. She indicates that she has discussed the role of the nurse at length with her father and other professionals. She is well aware of her ability and believes strongly in her own ideas. As a student she consulted the faculty, learned what the academic expectations of the faculty were, and produced accordingly while maximizing the experiences she felt she needed for the future. She became a specialist in first completing the faculty's requirements, then ignoring the faculty and forming her own education.

The prognosis for Francine's future and the future of the profession is good. Despite Francine's problems with intimacy as revealed by the tests, she can form in-depth relationships when she chooses. She has two close friends in the class who resemble her in intelligence and independence. She is engaged to a physicist who is finishing his doctoral work. She thinks they complement each other: she likes to be active and he prefers to be more passive and thoughtful. The nursing profession will certainly benefit from Francine's contributions.

Janice: A Nonacademic Dropout

Janice, like Francine, is pretty and bright and comes from an upper-middle class family involved in health care professions. Janice's father is a physician, her mother a nurse. She too went to college and studied biology for 2 years before entering nursing school. Here the resemblance stops. Janice lacks self-confidence and is still in the process of discovering her identity and establishing her goals. She falls into the Type I (modal) category on the 16 P.F.; she does not differ on the scales from the standard sample of college women. But Janice is a dropout.

She has the intelligence to complete the educational requirements and is not especially neurotic. Why did she leave? The primary reason was her conflict with the faculty and administration. The faculty was displeased with her behavior and attitude. She picked nursing for instrumental reasons; nursing represented future independence and the chance to obtain a good job. She was never fully comfortable in the student role. In high school she preferred social life to making good grades. Because of this she was turned down by the private institution of her choice in spite of her high scores on the entrance tests, and she went to a state university. At the state university she had a good time and received good grades, but felt that she had no direction. The courses were sometimes interesting, sometimes boring, but she did not see any relevance for the future in what she was learning. She considered medical education as a career but decided it was too long a program and involved too much work, both during school and after graduation.

The alternative was nursing, and she entered a school that she and her mother thought would give her a good education. In view of her background and college work, it is surprising that she picked a diploma school. Her rationale for the choice was that it would provide her with more practical experience in nursing than a B.S.N. program. She was tired of abstract knowledge and thought it would be easy to pick up the extra year needed for the B.S.N. if she decided to stay in nursing.

This "if" makes her unique. She is not like 80% of nursing students who enter nursing because "they always wanted to be a nurse." Unlike Francine, Janice is still not sure this is the field for her. She came into nursing education with the idea that she would try the role on for size. She had always enjoyed her contacts with the hospital. She had frequently accompanied her father at his work and had worked part time at hospitals during high school and college.

With this background, she felt that nursing deserved investigation, but she was not yet ready to make a career choice.

Her psychological tests indicate that she has some problems with her identity but that they are within normal limits. She is not neurotic, although she is still fighting some family battles. Her 16 P.F. scores show her to be low on anxiety, high on tough poise, high on extraversion, and very high on independence. This indicates a socially outgoing, enterprising, decisive, aggressive, and self-directing person. On the Identity Scale she scores high on autonomy within social limits, feels comfortable in groups, and has a positive evaluation of self.

However, she is experiencing career diffusion and has problems with emotional expressivity. Family dynamics may be the source of this conflict over the choice of nursing. When answering the question, "The part of nursing that has greatest appeal for me is—," she replies, "I don't know—ask my mother." When replying to the stem, "My chief aim in life is—," she states, "to be free." To the stem, "If my mother could change, I would want her to—," she answers, "not pressure me so much." To the stem, "My mother—," she comments, "does not really understand what I feel." To the stem, "If I weren't going to be a nurse, I would—," she answers, "fly to the moon, be free, be an astronaut." To the stem, "When they try to get me to be like my mother, I—," she says, "scream!" To the stem, "Nursing is—," she answers, "a plot to get me to do something I never really intended to do." From these statements we infer that she is not happy with the career she has chosen, is still tightly tied to her mother, and is not happy with this close relationship. Indeed, she might not have chosen nursing as a career; it may have been chosen for her by her mother, who apparently derives satisfaction from nursing.

Rebellion against parental pressure and uncertainty about career choice are typical of late adolescence. Why, in this case, did failure result? The problem seems to come from the fact that Janice worked out her rebellion against her mother on the faculty, and was overt about her lack of commitment to the field.

She certainly was no faculty favorite. She developed many ways of hoisting her instructors by their own petards. She carried out assignments to the letter, ignoring the spirit, thus horrifying the faculty member who had not considered the consequences of a literal interpretation of her remarks.

When assigned to do a complete social history on a child as a public health project, she interviewed both child and mother, not in the clinic but at their home, and included the extended family system. Janice's action was within the province of a public health nurse. However, no one had ever completed the assignment this way before, and the faculty was upset because the girl went into a very rough neighborhood and did not return for some time. Also, her actions could be considered a breach of confidentiality since she had infringed upon the patients' right to privacy. Nevertheless, she had completed the assignment and had done an excellent job, much better than the official social worker's report covering the same material.

Janice irritated the faculty in another way. She could pass tests without listening to the lectures. A reading list and a set of topics were sufficient, so she frequently cut lectures. This was ultimately her undoing. Her name was brought up again and again in faculty meetings because of her unorthodox response to assignments. Finally it was noted that she attended few classes and, although she had participated in the necessary clinical experiences, she was woefully lacking in attendance at lectures.

An old rule stated that students were not allowed to miss more than a certain number of hours of didactic material. The faculty seized on this, invoked the rule, and told Janice that she would be suspended if she missed three more hours of class. Janice obligingly came down with a strep throat, missed more than her three hours, and was suspended. She could have petitioned for reinstatement, and since she was an excellent student she probably would have been allowed to continue. However, she was enraged by the attitude of the instructors and by what she considered the unfairness of the situation. She did not bother appealing, but became a nonacademic dropout.

How did Janice progress through the developmental stages? She entered in Stage II, negative/independence. Her mother was her role model for nursing, and although she trusted her enough to try the field, Janice was already questioning when she entered nursing school. Her rebellion was overt and clever. She frequently did her assignments well, but in such a way that it pointed up the faculty's ineptness in planning the educational experience. The system could not withstand such overt rebellion. Janice found no role models in school who would help her find socially acceptable limits for her questioning. Her classmates were frightened by the overtness of Janice's rebellion, so Janice had no peer group for support.

Her future prognosis is good. She is a basically healthy person with many assets, but her future career will not be nursing. In many ways that is nursing's loss. Her ingenuity would have helped the profession.

Mary and Meagen: The Neurotic Road to Success and Failure

Mary and Meagen are similar in their backgrounds, appearance, and personality patterns. They differ only on cognitive factors. Meagen has the intellectual ability to complete her education but is not an outstanding student. Mary is exceptionally bright. Mary succeeds and Meagen fails.

All our instruments substantiated that both students are neurotic. They are both Type II, the neurotic introvert, on the 16 P.F. They score high on the anxiety and neurotic defense scales and low on the leadership scales. They both picked nursing for "expressive reasons." They considered nursing to be good preparation for marriage and expected nursing to provide them a great deal of personal satisfaction. According to the 16 P.F., both are introverted, liable to depression, agreeable, passive, and appear to be group-dependent.

Mary and Meagen are also similar on the Identity Scale. They are confident in their career choice, but have a poor self-image and experience problems with groups, autonomy, and trust. The sentence completion test indicates that both students think nursing will save them from their bad feelings about themselves and their fear of the environment. Both have problems with parents whom they consider overdemanding and cold. Both feel they are not living up to their mothers' expectations; can never be like their mothers, although they try; and wish their mothers were less nervous. They both view their fathers as cold and remote.

They are not twins, but each comes from a lower-middle class family and is the oldest daughter with many siblings. Both took a great deal of responsibility for raising their younger siblings because the mother was ill during their childhood. Both girls are unattractive, but this is largely their own choice. They are not pretty because they are heavy and have poor posture and grooming. Their poor self-conception clearly translates into an unattractive self-presentation.

Faculty members think Mary is terrific, although they do wish she were not so anxious and would lose some weight. However, she resembles their ideal student. Her assignments are always on time and completed to perfection. She absorbs all criticism and tries to correct any problem pointed out to her. Despite her anxiety, she is good with patients and can control her feelings with patients. Many faculty members take an interest in her and try to "bring her out of herself" so she could enjoy the learning experience.

How did Mary progress through the stages of socialization? She entered in Stage I and appears to have remained there. Psychotherapy helped her with family problems, but she refused to question the school or her career in nursing. She was committed to being a nurse and to the faculty's view of the nurse. The attitude that nurses must be perfect or risk patients' lives fits in with Mary's view that she has to strive for outer perfection or face her inadequacies.

After graduation, she worked for the hospital where the school was based. She was a good bedside nurse, but became upset and, as it turned out, incompetent when promoted to a position of control and responsibility. She subsequently resigned because she decided she did not like the administrative parts of nursing, and returned to school to receive her B.S.N. She did this easily and well and is now back at work in the hospital as a bedside nurse. She thinks that this is where she belongs and she is undoubtedly right. Within a well-structured context she is an excellent nurse. She is still afraid of making decisions and is deferent to authority. She has become a good handmaiden to the physicians on her unit.

Meagen, with similar personality traits and problems, is in trouble. She is not as bright as Mary, and emotional problems frequently interfere with her ability to retain and apply material correctly. She is not a favorite of the faculty. She lacks Mary's obvious brightness, so her anxiety and indecision are irritating. No one becomes involved with her and tries to make her feel less anxious about her performance. Indeed, several faculty members scolded her in view of her classmates. The faculty became alarmed by her level of anxiety and tried to see whether she was clinically safe and could function with this emotional burden. When she did poorly in one medical-surgical area, she became very upset. She did not think that she could take the stress and strain of the nursing responsibility. Although just on probation and not suspended, she withdrew. She did not return, although the faculty indicated she could if she so desired.

In terms of Meagen's progress through the stages of socialization, she too entered in Stage I, dependence, and stayed there. Unfortunately, she did not find anyone she could depend upon. No one viewed her as having enough talent to be a worthwhile investment of time and energy. This reinforced her negative self-perception. When her self-fulfilling prophecy came true and she did poorly, she took it as a sign that she was too incompetent to become a nurse. Meagen's emotional problems combined with a limited cognitive ability to produce failure. Her intelligence was adequate for functioning, but was inhibited by emotional problems. Mary's emotional problems were equally severe but her superior cognitive ability kept her functioning. Both students needed help to function well.

Stephanie: A Rebel With a Cause

Can a student with the normal identity problems of late adolescence, including rebellion against family and society, survive nursing education? Yes, provided she learns well how to con the faculty (Olesen and Whittaker, 1968); outright rebellion is frequently the road to nonacademic attrition.

Stephanie did not bother conning the faculty. When she entered a diploma nursing school, she was in search of a mother figure to help her understand and come to peace with herself and her problems. During the first 6 months she tried to identify with two of the younger, more "with it" instructors, but became disillusioned when they would not support her in one of her diatribes against the administration. She was a young woman with many pluses. She was intelligent, energetic, and attractive. She was also rebelling against her passive mother and her authoritarian father. The oldest of nine children, she has no memory of ever considering another profession. Nursing to her has always represented the royal road to the good life. Not just because it was a way out of the poverty into which she was born, but because of its nurturing and caretaking values. She thought that if she became a nurse everyone would then think she was a good person and, indeed, by tending the sick she would become a good person.

Despite her bond with the younger faculty members, her dependency needs were well hidden from both faculty and herself. She appeared to be an independent, critical, and demanding young woman. Personality tests showed assertiveness, poise, creativity, high anxiety, and great uncertainty about her identity.

Stephanie's first year was relatively calm. There was some grumbling among the administrators when she organized her peers for numerous protests, but she was considered more of a leader than a deviant.

The first 6 months of her clinical work changed this. The faculty stopped viewing her as intelligent and rebellious and began thinking of her as a menace. She had overt and angry breaks with the young instructors who had been her mentors. It was apparent that she had reached our model Stage II, resistance. She was comfortable with procedures, techniques, and the knowledge base of the field. She read widely and enjoyed taking on the instructors and challenging them on facts, theories, and techniques. This was the bane of some of the younger instructors who, just beginning their teaching career, were no match for her.

She was labeled a troublemaker and the faculty organized against her. A universal technique was developed and employed. Whenever she questioned or challenged an instructor, her attitude was criticized. The faculty asked her why she wanted to challenge and show off. Despite this warfare, she survived the medical-surgical experience and moved on to the specialized courses. The cold war escalated when she antagonized a newly appointed department chairperson who was too new to withstand any challenge. Stephanie viewed this chairperson as the authority figure against whom she could rebel and win, thus resolving some of her own unfinished psychological problems. The chairperson had not volunteered to serve as a target for a student's mental health, and went to the school director with the implicit ultimatum — the student leaves or I resign.

The peer group interceded and exerted pressure on Stephanie to be less rebellious. They pointed out that sometimes it was necessary to go along with the faculty whether one thought they were right or wrong. The other students were in Stage III interactionally and used each other to try on appropriate role behaviors. They urged Stephanie to do the same. A stormy session with the school director, who supported the chairperson and pointed out that a rebellious nurse could kill patients, reinforced the message. If Stephanie wanted to stay in nursing she first had to graduate, and this she could only do if she exhibited a less rebellious attitude.

This made her angry. She described the school, faculty administration and her classmates as a pack of hypocrites. She also reconsidered nursing as a career. She chose to continue despite the hypocrisy and did become quieter.

She graduated with excellent marks but no honors. The faculty had been too bruised by their encounters with her to vote her honors. Indeed, she almost did not graduate from the diploma school. At the graduation ceremony, each graduate was to wear a professional uniform she had selected as appropriate for her new situation. Stephanie's choice was a pink pantsuit—it was a costume before its time, and she and the school director had another go-around. She finally walked down graduation aisle in someone else's dress—but not without protest.

Upon graduation, she married and embarked on a career in nursing at the hospital where she had studied as a student. She became active in the union and quickly became known throughout the institution as an excellent nurse and a firebrand. In the meantime she continued her education for the B.S.N., graduating in record time by manipulating course sequences and placement tests. These manipulations created a pitched battle with the authorities, and the chancellor of the university had to intervene with the Nursing Dean for Stephanie to graduate. Despite completing both a diploma and a B.S.N. program, Stephanie was still in Stage II rebellion and ready to fight the field.

Shortly after receiving her B.S.N., her husband was transferred to another city. There she found a job in a health clinic and shortly thereafter was offered an opportunity to set up a new clinic in another neighborhood. She enjoyed this job. Since the new clinic was in a neighborhood with limited resources and multiple problems, racial and economic as well as health-related, no one tried to take from her the authority needed to run the clinic. After 2½ years the clinic was doing so well that state and federal agencies asked to inspect it. The success of the clinic led to an attempt at takeover by the medical establishment. Stephanie, however, was now not only a fighter but a sophisticated politican and, by maneuvering titles, kept control. She was now in Stage IV, interdependent, and identified with the profession. She could listen to the views of others but made her own decisions.

When her husband again transferred back to their home town, she returned to the hospital where she had previously worked. The institution offered her a good job with high status and a good salary, but she lasted only 3 months. In that rigid and authoritarian institution she felt she was back to square one. She did not try to lead a rebellion this time but considered her options and returned to school for her Master's degree. Again she manipulated the system and graduated in record time, but this time no one viewed her as a trouble maker. She still thought some of her actions were hypocritical, but she had made her peace with expediency and accepted the fact that sometimes one must tolerate unpleasantness. As a result, she enjoyed her experience in graduate school. With her Master's degree, she obtained a job as a member of a health care evaluation team which investigated the city's health care delivery system. Her critical, questioning mind and her ability to debate alternatives were assets to the team, and she was considered for promotion to project director.

How did this rebel, who finally became professional, proceed through the stages of professional socialization? The faculty was no more comfortable with her dependency than with rebellion. Although Stephanie had some Stage III peer experiences in diploma school, she graduated in Stage II rebellion and remained in that stage through her first work experience and her B.S.N. education.

Her progress to Stage IV apparently took place because, with no authoritarian superstructure, she and her colleagues formed a group that provided support for their decisions at the clinic. Since she could bring in consultants to help with various aspects of the clinic (such as budget planning, lobbying the local and federal governments for support, etc.), she did not feel adrift but rather in control. Consultants were her role models and her staff was a peer group and support system. Therefore, in an impossible job that no one else would touch, she arrived at Stage IV, interdependence.

NOTES

1. The materials from which test case studies were drawn are the numerous tests given entering students in conjunction with the HEW grant project (1974). These test results have been augmented by interview material and, in some cases, therapist's notes. Names and some details in the individual's lives have been changed to protect confidentiality. The tests are summarized in Appendix C.

Part IV

BUILDING A
PROFESSIONAL IDENTITY

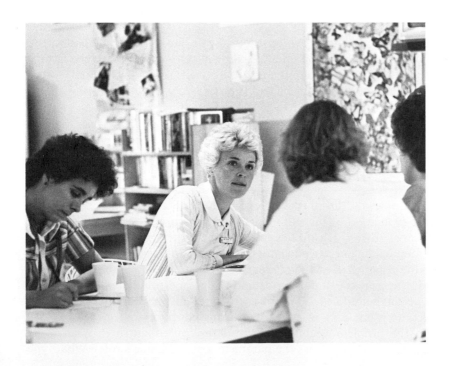

Chapter 10

FOUR STRATEGIES FOR CHANGE

At first glance, basic nursing education seems to have all the components necessary to produce a professional nurse. Knowledge and skills are evaluated throughout the educational experience. All would-be practitioners must pass licensing examinations. An apprenticeship program exposes students to controlled learning experiences, allows time for professional role testing, and enables students to practice professional work. Students can interact and identify with existing role models. Many schools have dormitories that help encourage student peer culture. This provides students with the strength and support to resist authority and a safe and understanding haven for expressing resentment and frustration. The peer group is a resource for ideas on how to handle problems; it provides input, feedback, and support.

These structures should provide students with a curriculum and an environment that allows them to develop cognitive skills and to integrate the professional role into their self-concept, but these hoped-for results have not taken place. What is missing? What went wrong? Why are graduate nurses not more comfortable with their roles? Why do large numbers of nursing students drop out? Why do many new graduates drop out in their first year? Why are many practitioners disillusioned, and many educators confused, about the definition and evaluation of the different educational programs?

The most obvious reason for these discrepancies is that the reality of the field propounded by nursing educators and leaders does not necessarily correspond to the experience of the student or staff nurse. Once the student has graduated, the clear-cut definition of knowledge and role boundaries learned in school becomes muddied. New nurses find that hospital administrators have role expectations not acknowledged by nursing educators.

Thus the problem begins with the definition of nursing: What is its knowledge base? What defines the parameters of the nurse's role? What type of health care decisions can she make? Are her functions autonomous, or are they dependent upon the physician's constant directives? These questions are not easy to answer because nursing is not only "churning for change," it is just plain churning. There is no unifying theoretical stance that can organize the profession. Indeed, there are not just two or three competing camps but a multitude of approaches, none definitive. A popular, if not unified, theoretical stance in nursing emphasizes practical matters over theoretical concerns. The question often asked when nursing and its problems are discussed is, "Who needs theory?"

THE IMPORTANCE OF NURSING THEORY

Greenwood (1972) chose a broad definition of a professional role and identified five elements of a profession: possession of a systematic theory, recognition by society of the profession's authority, community sanction, shared ethical codes, and possession of a culture (see Chapter 2). Systematic theory was listed first because the other attributes depend upon a theoretical base that defines the limits of the professional role for professionals and nonprofessionals.

Wang and Watson (1977) point out that nurses have been so preoccupied with functions (which change with time and circumstances) that they have given too little attention to conceptualizing the stable aspects of the nurse's role in terms of goals and intellectual focus. Simms (1977) states: "Nursing has been in the throes of seeking recognized professional status. In order to do this, nurses must prove that they have met the requirements of society with demands of the profession; i.e., autonomy, distinctive expertness, and control over practice and education." This distinctive expertness depends upon a theoretical stance that delimits the profession's knowledge base.

Nursing has been trying to define its theory and the nurse's role limits since nurses first tried to throw off the traditional role of nurturing and to become professional. In the 1970s, with the advancement of nurses in terms of recognition and salary, many educators turned their attention to defining and creating nursing theory.

Where does nursing theory stand today? This section contains a review of the literature on nursing theory, and analyzes the suggestions for establishing a theoretical base in nursing.

Leininger opened the University of Colorado's 1969 conference on "The Nature of Science in Nursing" by pointing out that there may be no single theory, model, or conceptual framework that would make nursing a legitimate professional field. Indeed, a search for such an answer is an exercise in magical thinking, and is highly unrealistic because any scientific discipline has multiple concepts, theories, constructs, models, and conceptual frameworks. Leininger coined the term "ethnoscience" to describe what she considered the proper approach to knowledge in nursing. Ethnoscience is "a systematic descriptive documentary study of phenomenon through the eyes, ears, and thoughts of the people in their situation. The nurse researcher using the ethnoscience method carefully and systematically could collect empirical data about concrete nursing situations from the subjects' viewpoint or frame of reference."

This may be a good way to start a research project, but it is not a stance that allows the individual to define the knowledge base, establish role limits, or set priorities among tasks. Indeed, as Schlotfeldt (1975) points out, this is an example of the task approach that nursing has always used, and suggests:

> To obtain verified nursing knowledge, the focus of inquiry must be primarily on persons served, rather than on practitioners and their characteristics, on specific sets of tasks in which practitioners engage at any point in time, or on the cost-benefits deriving therefrom. Professionals in nursing need to be concerned primarily with the knowledge of their practices, namely, its formulation and structure, its transmission through discourse, its application in practice, and its continuous advancement, refinement, and restructuring through scientific inquiry.*

Schlotfeldt's answer to this problem is to conceptualize nursing as:

> . . . the application of knowledge (science) and utilization of a variety of strategies with the goal of stimulating man's health-seeking behavior . . . . Following this scheme, the focus of nursing research designed to advance nursing science is on man's health-seeking behaviors—physiological, psychological, social, voluntary and involuntary, conscious and preconscious or subconscious, individual and group.**

This broad-based conceptual scheme does indeed solve the problem inherent in mere categorization of tasks, but leaves nursing with a data base that looks much like that of the applied social scientist.

Perhaps a systematic review of the definitions of theory and concepts and an examination of how nursing theory and theorists fit into a model of theory development are necessary. Dickoff and James (1975) discuss theory development for nursing. They distinguish four levels of performance in theory construction:

> I. Naming; II. Correlating; III. Situation-relative which would be predictive; and IV. Situation-producing or prescriptive. The levels are named here so as to make somewhat clearer how one level is related to another. At level I, conceptualizations are made to isolate factors; then at level II, the isolated factors conceived as related are used to describe situations. The next level, III, con-

---

*From Schlotfeldt, R.M. 1975. The need for a conceptual framework. In Verhonick, P.J. (editor): *Nursing Research* 1st ed. Boston: Little, Brown and Co., p. 288.
**From Schlotfeldt, *Nursing Research*, p. 687.

ceptualizes relations between situations described. Finally, level IV conceptualizes modes of producing situations of a specified kind.*

The various nursing theories can be categorized according to the levels described by Dickoff and James.

Leininger's (1969) ethnoscience approach is a level I or level II theory, depending on whether the individual simply describes situations or begins to describe relationships between situations. Hadley's (1969) view, that nursing's primary *raison d'être* is "to prevent and/or reduce the tensions that occur in man as a result of the stresses attendant to his entrance into the health care system," is also level II, correlating stress with treatment. Kramer (1968), in describing role deprivation, operates at level I, isolating and naming certain variables. Her concept of reality shock (1974) is a level II theory. Here she correlates the two types of tasks confronting nurses in the hospital situation (bureaucratic and professional) with the finding that many newly graduated nurses leave the field after one year.

The traditional view of the nurse-physician relationship is a care-cure dichotomy in which the physician diagnoses the ills and the nurse takes responsibility for the care of the patient under treatment. This is a level I (naming) type of theory, although it does define some relationships between the two disciplines. Montag's view of differentiating nursing into technical and professional competence, a position now officially adopted by the ANA, also is a level I theory.

Schlodtfeldt's conception of nurses as health care providers could be viewed as a level II (correlating) theory since it conceptualizes relations between situations; and perhaps as a level III (situation-relative) theory in which research leads to prescriptions to promote health.

Other theorists subscribe to the well-care approach, and their theories could be viewed as leading to level IV (situation-producing) of theory development. The most notable theories are Roy's (1971) adaptation model and Rogers' holistic theory (1970).

Roy's model (based on Maslow's self-actualizing theory) constructs four human needs: (a) physical means, (b) self-concept, (c) role function, and (d) interdependence. Utilizing this scheme, the nurse can decide which of her patients' needs are predominant and can try to meet all four types of needs through her nursing care plan. Implicit in the model is a hierarchy of needs, with interdependence being the highest level. Also implicit are the assumptions that the nurse should attempt to ensure that all the needs of the patient are satisfied, and that the higher-level needs are most important since they represent healthier functioning.

*From Dickoff, J., and James P. 1975. Theory development in nursing. In Verhonick, P.J. (editor): *Nursing Research* 1st ed. Boston: Little, Brown and Co., p. 324.

Roy's model is a useful conceptual scheme for organizing nursing data, but presents problems when applied to the everyday ward situation. Wagner (1976) asked graduate students to assess Roy's model in a variety of hospital situations. A standardized questionnaire that had been designed to test Roy's concepts was used, but students found it difficult to relate the questions to the exact part of Roy's model. Further, although they thought the model was a good framework for ordering a variety of observations, they found it difficult to implement. The students thought that the concepts were not useful in an intensive care setting and that it would take considerable dedication, education, and personal commitment to this model to make it functional in most nursing service situations.

Rogers' (1970) theory postulates a conceptual model of individuals that provides a framework for nursing inquiry. According to this scheme, each human is a unified system that cannot be understood except as a whole and in the complementarity of this relationship to the environment. Health problems, Rogers asserts, cannot be separated from the world's social ills. For Rogers, the notion of studying human social behavior, physiological behavior, or psychological behavior would not be appropriate for the investigator seeking to advance nursing knowledge because this approach does not address the role of the environment. Rogers, more clearly than Roy, proposes a level IV (situation-producing) theory because it has a complete view of the human condition and has (at least implicitly) an organizing construct — the individual's propensity for health. As such, it can be viewed as a situation-producing theory that clearly indicates which nursing tasks should take priority.

Unfortunately, Rogers' theory is no more practical than Roy's model. As useful as it might be in organizing knowledge in the abstract, Rogers' theory is of little use in the daily world of the intensive care staff nurse. Rogers' examples are designed to show what nursing theory can do for its knowledge base and thus differentiate nursing from medical knowledge, but they do not differentiate the role of the nurse from that of the clinical psychologist, community psychiatrist, or social worker.

These health-oriented theories (which emphasize the social and psychological needs contributing to health or illness) share a basic problem: They do not gibe with the ANA's distinction between the technical and professional nurse. The ANA assumes that the nurse with an advanced degree has more ability to plan, make decisions, and deal with the health, social, and psychological problems of the patient, but this means that most of these skills would be wasted in areas such as surgery, intensive care, and possibly burns and trauma, where the primary emphasis is on utilizing technology to save lives.

These areas now represent the most challenging aspects of nursing. The split-second requirements of the work allow nurses autonomous judgment, free from both hospital regulations and physicians' surveillance. Implementing the ANA and other health care theories would destroy this autonomy. Or perhaps, as Flint and Spensley (1969) state, "The professional-technical categorization probably is not the most functional way to classify nurses, but it looks as if it is here to stay, although it may have caused more problems than it has solved.''

One issue is certain: Either health care theories must be revised to include this distinction, or the distinction must be more carefully examined and revised to fit into health care theory. In any case, nursing presently has no theoretical stance or set of theoretical stances to give it a definite knowledge base. As such, it lacks one of the prime requisites for becoming a profession.

In view of this, it is rather disappointing that Dickoff and James (1975), after their excellent job in categorizing levels of theories, stated that the critical spirit in the question, ''Who needs theory?'' is a theoretical stance in and of itself. They suggest that nursing can borrow the questioning attitude of systems theory and can cultivate a spirit of knowledge for nursing, that would be more fruitful approach than the barren search for a body of knowledge specific to nursing.

Open-mindedness is an appealing quality for nurses, and indeed for all professionals. However, it does not solve the basic problem. If nursing is to become a true profession, it must meet the definitions of a profession. It must have an agreed-upon knowledge base and autonomy to make independent decisions within that knowledge base. A spirit of inquiry cannot provide this, nor can it differentiate between the roles of the professional and technical nurse. Both types of nurses would (the patients hope) have a sense of inquiry.

Simms (1977) summarizes the nursing problem: ''Many problems still exist. . . . Nursing's research is in its infancy and the results still too few. Definition of our distinctive knowledge remains hazy and this contributes to our lack of understanding of our role.''

Many nursing educators have suggested borrowing from other sciences (Johnson and Martin, 1958; McKay, 1969; Smoyack, 1969; Schlotfeldt, 1975), but so far, the borrowing is in the suggestion stage. Systems theory is frequently mentioned as the most appropriate model. It is not yet clear how systems theory fits into nursing care or how it would define nursing's knowledge base, set the priorities needed for professional judgment, or differentiate the medical, social, and psychological components of nursing.

It is no wonder that the entering nurse retreats in anguish after finding that there are bureaucratic tasks (filling out forms) as well as the physiological, social, and psychological tasks she was taught in school. She must rely on role models to guide her; she has not yet learned a conceptual scheme that allows her to analyze the situation and to decide which areas of the health care field are hers and hers alone. If for any reason her role models fail her, she leaves.

PROBLEMS CREATED BY NURSING CULTURE

Although nursing's educational structure is basically sound and aimed toward producing professional practitioners, it is short-circuited by the nursing culture. Throughout their education, students receive contradictory messages such as "If you are going to be a nurse, you must be perfect, never fail, and be a fully responsible individual; however, you are a handmaiden to the physician and must make sure you do as both the physician and the instructor tell you;" "Nurses must assess and make judgments; however, students must learn by rote, must never question or resist or they will be labeled troublemakers;" "If the nurse is not perfect, the patient may die;" "Nurses must appear self-confident for the sake of the patient's morale;" and "Nurses are the only ones who really understand the patient."

Regardless of how modern the curriculum or the type of teaching method, these age-old attitudes persist and continue to be communicated to the student. Indeed, as Mauksch (1963) points out, change rarely occurs at an even pace, and changes in rules and structures do not necessarily change attitudes. In 1974, Group and Roberts pleaded for nursing to free itself from the "ghost of the Crimea" (the tradition of obedience and subservience), to stop transmitting these values to students, and to stop labeling the questioning, bright students as troublemakers.

If one examines the professional self-concept in the Nightingale tradition, the root of the problem is easy to see. Nightingale defined the nursing role as handmaiden to the physician, and it has remained so. Handmaidens are not professionals, neither in the sociological definition used here nor in Stage IV (interdependence) in the socialization model.

Stein (1971) addresses this problem and describes the nurse who resorts to subterfuge by imparting knowledge to the physician without requiring acknowledgment of her opinion or power. Stein uses this dialogue as an example:

> Dr. Jones, this is Miss Smith on Ward Two. Mrs. Brown, who learned today of her father's death, is unable to fall asleep.

This message has two levels: Openly, it describes a set of circumstances (a woman who cannot sleep and who received word of her father's death this morning). Less openly, but just as directly, it is a diagnostic statement and recommendation; that is, Mrs. Brown is unable to sleep because of her grief, and she should be given a sedative. Dr. Jones accepts the diagnosis and replies to the recommendation by answering: "What sleeping medication has been helpful to Mrs. Brown in the past?" Not knowing the patient, Dr. Jones is asking for the nurse's recommendation about what sleeping medication should be prescribed. However, the question does not appear to be asking her for a recommendation.

Richards (1978) gives numerous examples of this situation. When a nurse must question a physician about treatment, it must be done in the kindest possible way, Richards states, otherwise her appeal will not be heard. The case of a 22-year-old pregnant woman with massive facial, head, and chest injuries is cited. The nurse recognized the severity of the injuries and wanted an obstetric consultation to see if the baby could be saved. However, she was too tact-ful, the resident did not receive her message, and a neurosurgeon was ordered instead. When the neurosurgeon could not be located, the resident called a chest surgeon who responded to the nurse's request and summoned an obste-trician. He performed a stat cesarean section to produce a stillborn baby. Richards asks whether the baby might have been saved if the physician had concentrated on the infant since it was evident that the mother was mortally wounded. ''What had gone wrong in this doctor-nurse game? The penalties of failure are severe. The nurse had made her recommendation without appearing to, but the doctor had refused to accept it.''

It is difficult to imagine any other two professional groups engaging in the dialogues described by Stein. Subservience and professionalism—the latter demanding judgment and the ability to put judgment into action—are anti-thetical. The nursing culture, internalizing such powerful contradictions, is bound to have trouble defining its role and educating neophytes.

Throughout her education a nurse is trained to play this doctor-nurse game. She is given two messages: the first states that the physician is omni-scient and any recommendation from her might be insulting to him, leaving her open to ridicule; the second implies that she is important to the physician, has much to contribute, and is obligated to make these contributions. The paradox is that when her good sense tells her to make a recommendation, she is not allowed to communicate it. Her solution is the doctor-nurse game, com-municating without appearing to do so.

These role conflicts are inherent in the existing nursing culture. The requirements for a subservient, dependent demeanor must be reconciled with the demand for perfection and a fear of killing a patient. How can one be sub-servient and totally responsible at the same time? The problem is the patient's ill health, and the nursing norm states that nursing care, if perfectly done, can rectify this problem. The danger of error has some basis in reality, and nursing instructors become protectors as they watch student behavior to assure clinical safety. Unfortunately, a necessary precaution becomes a straightjacket, demanding that all student behavior be monitored and assuming that all error is equally dangerous.

Until very recently, nursing faculties reviewed all student experiences because they contributed to professional learning. If such elaborate efforts must be made to protect the helpless patient from the learning student, the stu-dent can only conclude she is, for some unfathomable reason, a congenital hazard to the very people she wants to help. The result is an environment in which students feel constricted and spied upon and learn to present to the fac-ulty what the faculty wishes to see rather than what the students really feel or think (Olesen and Whittaker, 1968). Ironically, in an effort to produce only the highest quality nurse, nursing education drives out of the field the students most likely to become true professionals. The system, as it is presently constituted, is self-defeating. Students who are more assertive and more tolerant of their own aggression leave the program, while more anxious and neurotic students complete their education.

Instructors have the same problem as students. In *Silent Dialogue* (Olesen and Whittaker, 1968), students commented that their instructors were still young and inexperienced, thus incapable of giving them much practical experience. Alutto and others (1971) noted the propensity of the baccalaureate graduate to forsake practicing for teaching when confronted with the bureaucratic systems. Miller (1977) observed that nursing schools are prone to hire their own graduates, which perpetuates whatever subcultural norms exist.

Could Kramer's finding be another instance of the nursing culture undermining the structural system? Surely good professional training stresses different approaches to problems. Most students understand this abstractly but have great difficulty applying these approaches to practice.

Reality shock results from faculty expectations of obedience and perfection in students. Regardless of changes in the curriculum, these expectations force the student to conform. If students are told to try alternatives, implicit in the message is "find the *right* alternatives" (Torrance, 1964). The culture persists in aligning all knowledge with caretaking and all error with death. For example, in *Silent Dialogue*, Olesen and Whittaker (1968) report that a classroom instructor considered a student to be clinically unsafe because of a poor showing on a math test. In other words, students were to be kept off wards until they passed the test. The students' anxious response to this announcement was gratifying to the instructor. Unfortunately, this is *not* a hypothetical or isolated example. In 1974, I found one math instructor terrifying students by screaming, "If you add that way on the ward, your patients will die!"

The point is not that excellence should not be required, but that an educational system making such demands should support students wrestling with the responsibility of health care. Fox (1957) points out that medical schools recognize that their students must master three types of uncertainty. The first stems from self and imperfect mastery of available knowledge; the second, from the limitations in current medical knowledge; and the third, from the difficulty of distinguishing between personal ignorance and limitations in the field. Nurses, confronted with a more limited data base, are warned that they must know it perfectly. These cultural pressures and the absence of a theoretical knowledge base make it difficult for a nurse to become professional, even in a perfect environment with all the necessary structural elements.

PROGRAMS AIMED AT
SOLVING THESE PROBLEMS

Nursing seems to be caught in Catch-22. The individual most capable of professionalism—the bright, questioning, and aggressive female who could change the outer structure and the inner symbolic culture of the group—is the individual most likely to be factored out. The stage for testing limits and establishing self-autonomy and initiative is, if not missing, negligible and hidden. If the competent individual insists on experiencing this stage, she will be pressured to conform or leave.

Nursing researchers have not discussed this stage and its role in the socialization of nurses. Kelman's (1967) theory on socialization and attitude change cites the components of compliance, identification, and internalization, but Kelman does not mention resistance as a part of socialization. Kramer, in detailing Kelman's theory, does not comment on the omission of this stage.

Although educators have not recognized the need to encourage or support students through Stage II, resistance, and have not searched for ways to include it in the educational system, they have been concerned about the high incidence of attrition. Successful attempts have been made to reduce attrition within the educational system and during the first year after graduation. Further, the philosophies of almost all schools reflect a concern with professionalism, and their goal is to produce a truly independent practitioner.

Four programs are examined: the first two attack the problem of attrition. The third illustrates a change in structure and the fourth a change in the physician-nurse relationship.

Solution 1: Transforming Nursing Dropouts to Drop-ins

In a school with a historical 40% to 50% attrition rate, Rubin and Cohen (1974) investigated the effectiveness of brief group psychotherapy sessions for underachievers combined with a remedial basic skills program in reducing the attrition rate. (An underachiever was a student with a grade point average lower than a "C" and whose academic predictor scores indicated the ability to perform adequately.) The psychotherapy or "motivational" groups used Roth's techniques (Roth, 1963, 1970; Roth and Puri, 1967), demonstrating that confrontation group counseling compels the student to look at herself as an active and causal force and enables the failing students to solve emotional and academic problems. Roth thought the typical underachiever's problems stemmed from how he or she learned the role of work in our society. Some students become motivated to fail and remain childlike and dependent rather than renounce a comfortable lifestyle for independence and maturity.

In the psychotherapy group, peer as well as therapist pressure can be exerted on any individual persisting in failure-motivating behavior. The group process discourages those rationalizations previously used to explain and justify failure. Relationships that develop among group members help individuals accept the responsibility for their fate. The group experience also helps free students from fears of and dependence on authority figures. Combined with tutoring in basic skills, this program reduced the attrition rate to 21%.

Subsequent research (Cohen, 1974), funded by a HEW nursing demonstration grant, expanded the program to include undereducated overachievers (high-risk inner-city students with very low NLN aptitude test scores). An administrative edict to the school resulted in recruitment of inner-city students who, under usual circumstances, would have had no chance to enter nursing. Before entering, they were enrolled in a summer remediation program, which improved their basic language and math skills considerably. However, this group's NLN aptitude test scores were still not high enough to permit acceptance. Under administrative fiat these students were admitted as risk students and were included in the psychological intervention program designed for underachievers.

Again, the expanded program showed that underachievers responded well to brief confrontational psychotherapy. Much to the surprise of the director and staff, so did "overachievers," the high-risk students. As the director stated:

> It was a pleasant surprise to find that the treatment developed for one characterological program (the underachiever) also worked well with academically deprived students (summer risk), for whom it was never intended and who could be assumed to have very different needs. The [overachievers] were aspiring to educational goals for which they were not adequately prepared. Of those in the group who went without treatment, 93% failed (14 out of 15); those with treatment had an attrition rate of 27% (3 out of 11).

> The explanation can probably be found in the self-concept of the inner-city student, particularly in the view of self as learner. According to theory, the reason motivational groups work and break up long standing [habitual] patterns of nonwork is that the therapeutic method confronts the student with the fact of his having chosen nonwork as a defense mechanism. Typically, the underachiever blames others and the world for the problems and thinks that tomorrow—somehow, magically—the knowledge necessary to pass and succeed will arrive. A therapy which makes the student realize that only his choices and his efforts can do anything to improve the situation tends to crack the core of the problem. It is difficult to face a perceptive therapist plus a group of one's peers week after week with excuses such as "the library is too quiet."

> Motivational groups for the inner-city students utilized this confrontational technique to point out that students are active architects of their own fate, a realization which comes as a shock to them. While doubtless there is much that is real in their complaints, when therapy is effective they realize they have the ability to make their own choices regarding many of these matters and assume responsibility in their educational careers. The fact that their past schooling was deficient and they were unable to learn does not mean this situation has to continue. In some instances, rationalizing failure by crying "racism" is a defense of the same order as "the library is too quiet." When they begin to use, rather than hide from, the academic remediation offered,

and to view themselves as individuals who were behind but capable of catching up, their probability of success was enhanced.*

This program worked, but for reasons other than those the investigator cited. A more intensive analysis of the process was necessary.

Solution 2: Preventing Disillusionment and Attrition Among Graduates

Kramer (1974) originated and investigated an attrition prevention program for recent graduates. Using "anticipatory socialization," it endeavored to build into the educational program a process to make the student aware of the realities of practice and the strategies needed to cope with the bureaucratic structure while retaining the professional ideals. The original program included four phases:

Phase I: The Encounter. Phase I covered the first year and consisted of ten seminars held twice a month with groups of 15 or 16 students. Basically, each focused on attacking the professional values being learned in the remainder of the curricula. This deliberately produced a mild shock to accustom the student to differences between the nursing faculty's values and the practices that might go on in the reality of the hospital.

Phase II: Reidentification. Since students entered the educational program with higher bureaucratic loyalties than they would have at the end of the first year, after the nursing faculty had indoctrinated them with their professional values for a year, this phase allowed students to return to earlier values in order to promote an adaptive or "bicultural" blend. This blend would allow for appropriate choosing of the bureaucratic or professional mode. Students were encouraged to work during the summer as hospital aides and to discuss any hospital problems encountered during the seminar. They were also encouraged to find a role model to identify with—someone in the work environment who appeared at ease with both sets of values.

Phase III: More Conflict, but Hope. This phase's goal was to reestablish the professional goals and to encourage students to think creatively and broadly about system changes necessary for effective health care delivery. Conducted during the program's second year, it dealt with issues such as potential physician-nurse role conflict or support of colleagues, the nurse and the law, presentation of self in the work role, and evaluation of strategies in terms of accomplishments in work settings.

Phase IV: Affirmation. Phase IV—theoretical models useful in conflict resolution and role negotiation—took place during the third and last year of the program.

Certain themes were stressed throughout the program, unifying differences in the content and handling of the phases:

*From HEW Report. 1975. To facilitate learning by providing a multi-varied attack on the problem of attrition and staff-student relations. Cohen, H.A., principal investigator, p. 47.

1. If at first you don't succeed, keep trying.
2. People are unpredictable.
3. There are at least two alternatives.
4. Conflict is healthy and creative.
5. Work that is meaningful is of paramount importance.
6. Develop a tolerance for uncertainty.
7. Development of interpersonal competence in several social contexts is necessary for maximum effectiveness.
8. Learn to recognize when outside help and support is needed, and find someone who can provide it.

Although it did not significantly decrease the school's attrition rate, this program did reduce withdrawal after the first year and also promoted a high percentage of reentry into the profession later. Kramer states, "It appears that one possible effect of exposure to the program was a greater tendency to delay completion of the formal nursing education program until one had a chance to go out and look things over." (All but two of the 13 students worked as nurse's aides during the period before reentry.) Graduates of the program experienced less role deprivation than a similar control group from previous classes. There was less job turnover and fewer graduates left the field. Interestingly, the faculty viewed the anticipatory-socialization class as more resistive and feisty than the previous class. They were viewed as good nurses but troublemakers — bound for problems later because they were always asking questions.

Subsequently, an abbreviated anticipatory socialization program was given to new graduates experiencing the conflict between bureaucratic and professional values in their first jobs. Again, although the time allotted and the scope of this program did not compare with the original program, the seminars did appear to fill a need. The graduates subsequently reported less role conflict, less role deprivation, and were less likely to leave the field or the unit where they worked. Kramer views both programs as successful because they provided the student with an inoculative dose of future happenings. Students were exposed to the work organization, the differences between the school's explicit expectations and the working world's implicit expectations, and differences between local or bureaucratic and cosmopolitan or professional points of view, thus promoting biculturalism. In this case, it promoted the ability to live in the bureaucratic and professional culture.

Comparison of Attrition-Preventing Programs

Both programs cast light on the phenomena they studied and both reduced attrition rates. (Indeed, the HEW program worked for individuals not considered appropriate for the program's type of treatment.) Both programs gathered students in groups to discuss problems, to explore the problems, and to arrive at solutions.

The topics discussed by the groups differed markedly. For instance, there would be no point in discussing the future work role with failing students. However, the groups appeared to serve identical functions. They stimulated the individuals to think about the nursing role and the institution and to express negative feelings. Kramer's seminars actively promoted Stage II resistance and insisted that students question the dominant values. The motivational groups in my research channeled the students' self-destructive resistance into productive strategies. Both programs promoted group cohesion and the mutuality necessary for growth in Stage III.

The effect of the motivational groups on student resistance in the HEW-sponsored program was evident to the researchers. Early in the program it was apparent that the groups were expressing issues and feelings not usually dealt with by faculty and administration. Release of emotion combined with the rechanneling of energy into academic efforts effectively broke up the underachievement motive. The goals of this program were simpler than Kramer's; the students were encouraged to graduate, and concern about whether they would become independent practitioners or would remain in nursing after graduation was postponed. Kramer's program was aimed at producing fully functioning professionals who would exemplify Stage IV, interdependence. They would be bicultural and therefore able to use either bureaucratic or professional values when appropriate; they would know when to consult and when to use their own judgment.

Despite the more limited goals and a more disadvantaged group, follow-up data indicates that the students in my project arrived at a satisfactory level of Stage IV, interdependence. All students who graduated passed state board examinations (even though, in the case of risk students, this had not been anticipated by the faculty). The majority accepted positions at the school-affiliated hospital. All students remained in the field for at least one year. Over 80% had been promoted by the end of this year. The students expressed satisfaction with nursing and reported so to the project director.

They did not express any affection for the school or the research program. Both were still viewed as infringement on their autonomy. However, they came to realize that tolerance is necessary for survival in the professional world. This tolerance was extended to the bureaucratic structure. They were resigned to the older nurses who were sometimes irascible and to psychologists who did "strange" things for a living. As one student, who had been vocally angry about being required to attend motivational groups, stated at a post-graduate interview: "Well, I guess you have to earn a living like everyone else, and if that's the way you get your jollies, it's better than pulling the wings off of flies. At least I now have a job I like with a lot of bread, so I guess we can quit even."

Solution 3: Promoting Independence
via an Open Curriculum Structure

The third program was a structural solution designed to promote student autonomy and responsibility by giving students some control over their education. The "open curriculum" program was formulated so students could progress at their own speed. The school was on a nongraded pass-fail system, and students were allowed to repeat each examination up to three times if they failed to make the criteria of excellence the first time. All requirements were spelled out in great detail so students knew precisely what would be expected in each module or unit. Videotape material and detailed reading lists supplemented the lectures.

With these innovations, much of the traditional evaluation power of the faculty hands became impersonal and standardized. Students could choose to accelerate their studies, to extend them, or to go through the course in average time. An average time for a given module of learning might be 12 weeks; some accelerated students would finish in 8 weeks; others could take up to 16 weeks to finish. The students were responsible for completing all designated learning experiences (unlike some schools where absence might mean missing an experience) and could take proficiency examinations at any time. If a student did not pass the examination, it could be repeated the following week.

This system, with its built-in guarantee of student control over the learning experience, should have promoted student autonomy and initiative. However, it provided no support for the initial stage, dependence. The result was that students felt pressured into autonomous behavior without having the background to make them comfortable with that behavior. They did not trust the socializers who were demanding so much of them so quickly. When students and faculty were interviewed about their perception of problems in the system, both cited the time faculty members and students spent together as a major problem. The faculty thought that the program was terribly demanding and that the students required much individual attention. The students complained bitterly that the faculty did not have enough time for them. Were they talking about two different schools?

In view of the socialization process, this result makes sense. The students are confused and bewildered in the sea of knowledge and techniques, looking for guidance and structure. Instead, they are told to be their own navigators.

This system was established in a "commuter" school, which had few dormitories. Widely diverse living arrangements and differing time schedules made it difficult to form student study groups. The students started to compete with one another, feeling that the faculty demanded acceleration. One student stated: "Everyone says taking average time is all right, but you know if you do, the faculty think you are dumb. Also, if you don't keep up, you lose your friends because you won't be in the same classes."

Is a system designed to foster independence supporting dependency instead? The socialization process seems to encourage dependency by demanding too much, too soon. Students are not allowed to experience the necessary dependency, and since faculty does not control a good deal of the grading process in the first 2 years, students do not view faculty as objects of hostility and resistance. Indeed, the system appears difficult to resist. One student pondered: "There really is a bad competitive atmosphere in the school but no one really wants to talk about that. I guess it's [the students], not the faculty."

Students subtly let the faculty and administration know they were angry. One Christmas party given by faculty was bypassed by all but six (of 100) students. The others claimed they "lacked time"—an excuse students often heard from the faculty.

Significantly, at the end of junior year, when, according to the socialization scheme, they should be entering into Stage III, mutuality, these students reported a "burnt-out" feeling because they were deprived of the system of group support. Apathy set in and no one knew why. This apathy may be indicative of anger turned inward. Since it was difficult for students to expresss the resistance and anger of Stage II, and because the consistent interactions necessary for group formation were not available, the students have no channel for their energy. They take it out on themselves and soon feel "burnt-out and needing time off."

Many students respond by taking a break, utilizing time credits built up with accelerated courses so they will graduate, not early but on target. They retreat from school and the rat race. Usually they say they want to reevaluate their goals and their nursing career. When they return, they are prepared to act autonomously and enjoy senior-level courses. Interestingly, this school draws a large number of older students who have raised families and are now returning to school to prepare for a career. These students (comprising half the class) are the faculty's delight and are usually picked as outstanding students. They probably experience less trouble with the socialization process of this particular system because they enter less in need of support for Stage I, dependency.

Solution 4: Overcoming the Doctor-Nurse Game

Thomstad and others (1975) report on a project where a physician and a nurse began playing the doctor-nurse game by different rules. They were employed to work together in providing comprehensive primary care for a satellite clinic in an urban medical center. It was apparent to both that, if the project was to succeed, a more open system of communication and a peer rather than a hierarchical type of role interaction would have to develop.

As the clinic work progressed, they developed a new set of rules:*

*From Thomstad, B., and others. 1975. Changing the rules of the doctor-nurse game. *Nursing Outlook* 23:425.

Old Rules	New Rules
1. Medical care is more important than nursing care.	Good health care requires both good nursing care and good medical care.
2. The nurse can help the doctor as long as nobody knows about it, including the doctor.	The doctor and nurse are both there to help the patient and have to communicate directly and openly to do so.
3. The doctor knows more than the nurse.	Good doctors know more medicine than good nurses; good nurses know more nursing than good doctors.
4. If the doctor tells patients what to do, and they don't do it, it is the patients' fault. The doctor did his best.	If a health care plan is to be carried out, it must be worked out with the patient's needs, beliefs, and capabilities in mind.
5. Doctors are so busy that nurses may have to take over some of the tasks.	Many doctors do not like or know much about health care. Nurses are prepared in this, like it, and are usually better at it than doctors.
6. Good doctors rarely make mistakes and see to it that others do not either.	Everyone makes mistakes, but open communication between doctors and nurses minimizes them.

These new rules obviously give the nurse her own turf and data base. Note, for example, the new Rule 3: "Good doctors know more medicine than good nurses; good nurses know more nursing than good doctors." It is also implicit that the nurse has autonomy and ability to question and to make judgments on her own. The physician involved in this project did not evolve these new strategies and the new rules without considerable pain to himself.

Why were this nurse and physician successful in negotiating a new relationship? From a sociologist's perspective, there were many reasons. One reason was that both partners were true professionals and were less concerned with conventional career options and professional success than they were with interesting work. Role status needs were somewhat subordinated in favor of the overriding goal of good patient care to which they were both committed. The collaboration was effective, and the success of this project is evidence of this.

Less effective, however, was the integration of the project in the network of service organizations within which the project had to function. Professional reactions were particularly strong, perhaps because this was not just a one-stop play. It was invented, funded, and practiced to challenge the old game, goals, rules, and players. The government expected other agencies and institutions to follow this model.

As small as the project was, both the new system and the players threatened health care professionals. Other physicians expressed their dissatisfaction with the project and with the expanded nurse's role by labeling the physician a mental lightweight who could never finish anything. Nurses also reacted to the autonomy and refused to take the nurse in the project as a role model. Indeed, they stayed away from her, and emphasized the traditional handmaiden role. They thought the project nurse took on the added responsibility because of personal, not professional, reasons. The rumor circulated that the project nurse was in love with the physician, and that this love was unrequited. The inference was that she was a failure as a woman, even though she might be a success as a professional.

The implication of this article is that one of the problems in changing nursing roles is the nurse who may not want the power in professionalism because it means giving up traditional femininity. This internal problem may be more of a stumbling block to professionalism than the outside influence of the physician who prefers to keep the power base for himself and his colleagues.

CONCLUSION

Many nurses and nursing educators have tried to provide educational and remedial programs that promote independence and professional behavior among nursing students. But few, if any, understand the causes of nursing problems.

This chapter analyzed the problems with nursing theory and culture and with programs designed to promote professional growth. The problem with theory and culture still exists, although there is one example of a successful attempt to overcome the doctor-nurse game. Two of the structural programs, although applied to different populations and using different techniques, were successful because they provided a group process that allowed the students to progress through the stages of socialization.

The third program dramatically restructured its curriculum to allow students more flexibility and autonomy in their educational experience. This program was also successful, but the lack of support for Stage I tends to produce problems for some junior-year students.

The next chapter contains suggestions for changes in the educational system, utilizing these insights from the nursing literature and these programs.

Chapter 11

PROPOSED SOLUTIONS

The solutions proposed here are based on my conception of the underlying problems in the nursing profession: the lack of a theoretical system to delineate a unique body of knowledge, and the existence of a culture that prohibits autonomy for practitioners.

PROBLEMS STEMMING FROM
THE LACK OF A THEORETICAL BASE

An important dimension of the professional role is possession of a systematic theory and control over the knowledge base of the field (see Notes to Chapter 2). Many of nursing's problems can be traced to the fact that most of the conceptual schemes used to describe a nurse's function are what Dickoff (1975) describes as Level I (naming) types of theory.

The conceptual models in nursing, such as the professional/technical and care/cure, illustrate the approach of the semiprofessions (Simpson and Simpson, 1969). While these conceptual models may temporarily allow nurses professional activity—assessing patient needs, evaluating the total picture, and making health care decisions—neither model provides for future changes in the nurse's role, nor do they provide any assurance that the nurse's decisions will be enforced.

Technical versus professional is a distinction more meaningful to nurses than to the community or to other health care professionals. The care/cure model, in which the physician is in charge of curing the patient and the nurse has responsibility for the care of the patient, preserves the handmaiden status of the nursing role and ought not serve as a model. A theoretical approach must differentiate these two functions in such a way that the nurse's care role has autonomy and recognition. In other words, a nurse's decision should influence a physician's cure domain the same way the physician's cure decision influences the nurse's care plans.

As discussed in Chapter 10, the models and theories that have been proposed for nursing have inherent problems that their originators have not yet addressed. While these models and theories do provide nursing with knowledge that the physician does not have (psychological and sociological insights), they do not explicitly differentiate the nursing function from that of the applied social scientist, the clinical psychologist, or the social worker. Nursing can, indeed, make a valuable contribution to the health care field by bringing a psychological-sociological approach to patient care and by focusing on health rather than illness. However, they must not let their enthusiasm for newly found skills overshadow their fund of biological knowledge. Care for the physical needs of patients must remain the core of the nursing role.

A theoretical stance that defines the nursing role and its unique knowledge base would free nursing from the striving for perfection that contributes to the authoritarianism of nursing culture. Nursing does not yet recognize the uncertainty and limitations of the health care knowledge base. Medical students, as stated previously, are educated to deal with this uncertainty (Fox, 1957). Nurses are not. Nursing's proud tradition of getting the job done despite obstacles tends to blind nurses to the limitations of knowledge and skill. Even experienced practitioners idolize "super" nurse, the individual who can do everything and do it perfectly (Cohen and Orlinsky, 1977).

PROBLEMS STEMMING FROM
THE AUTHORITARIAN CULTURE

The lack of autonomy in nursing is apparent at all levels — student, practitioner, teacher, and administrator. The nursing student of the 1970s entered a system that was autocratic at the core. She could not indulge in even covert resistance for any length of time. The structural and cultural supports for resistance were almost totally stifled by the lack of opportunity for expression and by the strong sanctions against questioning and assertiveness.

Autonomy is also a problem for the faculty. Often faculty members have not resolved the conflicts of the professional nursing role. It is apparent from the literature that not too many educators have come face to face with their own professional role models (Williamson, 1972; Kohnke, 1973). Many are hired by their parent institutions immediately after completing their master's degree and re-create the problems they encountered as students (Miller, 1977). Most professional fields prefer a dissemination system, in which new graduates join other institutions and return to their own school (if at all) only after a number of diverse experiences.

At the administrative level, the problem becomes one of perception. Although nursing leaders generally perceive how authoritarian the medical and university establishments are, they do not perceive how authoritarian they are themselves, or how their insistence on error-free performance perpetuates problems with autonomy. Administrators in nursing think they support any change that will improve the status and educational system of nursing. They are willing to endorse programs aimed at changing the authoritarian and perfectionist attitudes of their staff, but few administrators see that their own authoritarianism causes problems.

The following cases illustrate this problem: One nursing director, well aware of her staff's rigidity and authoritarianism, sent the following memo to her staff: "You *must* not teach so authoritatively, you must teach nondirectively." A hospital director frequently admonishes his directors with: "You *must* not be so authoritarian with your staff."

Another important aspect of the authoritarian culture is the doctor-nurse relationship. Many nurses and educators have bridled at suggestions that the doctor-nurse game is still in effect and that nurses do not have control over their working environment. They cite the new nurse practitioner and assert that there is no longer any need to play such games and that autonomous roles for nurses do exist. Even a cursory look at recent nursing literature indicates that the doctor-nurse game is alive and well (Richards, 1978).

In our culture, human life is near the top of the hierarchy of values, so organizations that deal with human lives, such as law and medicine, are very rigidly structured. Indirect communication is an inefficient mode of transmitting information, but it supports and protects the organizational structure and the physicians' authority. Expanding medical horizons, however, mean that physicians' continuing expectations of doctor-nurse game interaction will be disastrous. The nurse must have the privilege of expressing her opinions and observations.

This authoritarian culture combined with the lack of a theoretical base prevents nursing from attaining professional standing. The remainder of this chapter contains suggestions for resolving these problems.

SOLUTIONS

A Universally Accepted Theoretical Stance

As with most situations, the first step to a solution is recognizing the situation and admitting that a problem exists. The 1969 ANA conference on theory and research was a good beginning, but its basic premise—that theory is necessary only for nursing research—illustrates the problem. As one established nurse-sociologist stated: "You cannot write another book about the nurse's role. We have been dealing with that problem since the 1940s and now the nurse-practitioner movement has solved it. Nurses should stop discussing what their role is and just get on and do it."

Unfortunately, the result of this would be the perpetuation of the task orientation of nursing. The numerous articles by young nurses (see *Supervisor Nurse* 1978 and 1979) reveal dissatisfaction with the field and problems in defining nursing roles and boundaries, and prove that the basic problem is not solved by nurse-practitioners. The first step, then, is an admission that there is a problem which cannot be either glossed over or argued out of existence.

The second step is doing something about it. Through its national organization, the ANA, nursing can organize the academic leaders in the field so they can unite and put the same type of energy into producing theoretical positions and models as they exhibited in their survey of the educational system in "Abstract for Action." This does not mean that there must be one single theory, but a consensus must exist as to the knowledge base the theories or models will conceptualize. There must be uniformity in terms of role description and establishing the priorities inherent in the role. Without this crucial underpinning to define the field's knowledge base, nursing—regardless of any structural revisions—will remain a semiprofession.

Reeducation of the Socializers

If the field is to change, the socializers must change—radically. Nursing educators must become less authoritarian and more capable of understanding and accepting their own and students' aggression. They must accept students' questioning of data and faculty. They must realize that they contribute to the problem and can be a major part of the solution. I concur with Hassenplug's (1977) view that one must:

> Help . . . these nurses strengthen their preparation, shift their accountability from physicians and institutions to clients, and become contributing members of their professional organization, whose goals include improvement of nursing practice and nursing education and greater say in the delivery of health care services. To do this we must embark upon a nationwide continuing education program designed to socialize or resocialize thousands of these nurses to the professional role.*

Most people are capable and willing to see authoritarianism in others and suggest changes; few are ready to see it in themselves and volunteer to change. The problem of authoritarianism is so deep-rooted in nursing that it has the strength of early group identifications involved in ethnic prejudice. If nursing is to change as a profession, the leaders within the group must come to grips with this authoritarianism and their lack of trust, which is not just a lack of trust of outsiders but of each other.

Birnbaum (1975) describes a group experience, which he labels "Clarification (C) Group," that ameliorates intergroup tensions. The program was originally designed to help ease racial and religious tensions by enabling individuals to understand and learn to deal with their own ethnocentrism.

*From Hassenplug, L.W. 1977. Nursing can move from here there. *Nursing Outlook* 10(4):436.

The C Group concentrates on three categories of questions: (a) Who am I in terms of my group identification? (b) How do others respond to me in terms of my group identifications? (c) How do I respond to others in terms of their group identifications; that is, what stereotypes and what generalizations do I make? Answering these questions facilitates insight into personal and interpersonal problems.

This type of seminar, run by the professional nursing organizations on the state or national level, could help resocialize nursing role models. In these seminars, the upper administration and faculty begin to see their impact on others and can learn to give and receive feedback. This must begin with upper administration and the leaders in the nursing field, because (as is evident to anyone who has tried to use organizational development programs to change managers' attitudes) the upper levels of administration must not only endorse the programs, but must themselves begin the process of change. If nursing administrators grant the faculty freedom to question the administration, the faculty will feel free enough to proceed to work through their problems of their own professional images. The administration can never grant this freedom until it realizes that it is part of the problem and that administrators' self-evaluation must be part of the solution. When administration and faculty have completed the process, they will be able to cope with the students' problems.

Another type of group approach to the faculty is Caplan's (1964) consultation methodology. Caplan describes the consultation process:

> [In] Consultee-Centered Case Consultation the problem relates to the staff's fears that they lack the skill, resources, or professional objectivity needed to deal with a particular problem. Hence the project or individual with whom they must cope is doomed. The consultant, by providing alternative solutions to the problem, alleviates the "doom" aspect that many knotty problems imply.*

This approach was used successfully in the HEW grant project, when administrative changes made the faculty feel the situation was hopeless. Caplan's "doom" (a feeling that the situation was impossible and impervious to human efforts) was felt everywhere. The faculty group met for 6 months (this time period was a function of the outer turmoil, not necessarily the professionalism of the faculty). At the end of the group sessions the faculty confronted the new administration with a manifesto detailing the support they needed to accomplish their jobs effectively. With this they had reestablished their autonomy and reaffirmed their professional identities. The experience of dealing with such an overwhelming problem was ultimately beneficial to all. Each group member felt more confident in professional encounters.

---

*From Caplan, G. 1964. *Principles of Preventive Psychiatry*. New York: Basic Books, Inc., p. 214.

Learning to Deal with Medical Uncertainty

Faculty members and administrators can benefit from learning the concept of medical uncertainty (Fox, 1957) and the techniques used in some medical schools to train neophyte physicians to deal with uncertainty. Faculty members should approach this topic with the student's self-concept in mind. Identification with an occupation or profession "ties up the loose ends" of the individual's identity and helps integrate all stages of development and the concepts of self that preceded each stage (Erikson, 1950). The work identification propels the adolescent into adulthood, and it is important that an individual maintain a positive self-concept during this process. Educators must realize that demands placed upon students and themselves for error-free performance affect an individual's personality and attitudes and can hinder the professionalization process.

Seminars can aid in teaching nurses to live with uncertainty, and help lessen the fear of a patient's death. After putting the problem of error in perspective, the seminars can focus on techniques useful in teaching students to deal with death as a potential consequence of treatment. Fox (1957) found that since the medical school he studied did not force-feed data but relied on broad technical topics, lists of references, and lectures from a number of viewpoints, first-year students felt overwhelmed and were appalled at their limited knowledge and skill. However, as students mastered the base level of knowledge and moved on, they perceived that some instructors were better than others, all had limitations, and sometimes the problem in diagnosis is based on the limitations inherent in medical knowledge.

Caplowitz (1961) suggests that when medical students enter their third year of education and are exposed to a greater number of faculty members who serve as role models, they become more willing to rely on their own critical judgment and become more adapt at evaluating the competence of faculty members. With this progression, they become increasingly capable of playing the role of physician. According to Caplowitz, this increasing capacity for judgment and its corresponding rise in professionalism is a function of the extended frame of reference.

Nursing students are also exposed to a variety of practitioners as they proceed through their educational specialties. However, they are frequently caught in a conflict between the faculty and practitioners, and are told by faculty to ignore what the practitioners are doing and instead listen to the faculty's instructions. The result of this is not to sharpen the critical faculties but to deaden the questioning process. Students will give faculty what they want—the "right" response—and not learn that alternative procedures exist. After several years of this the students are well-conditioned to believe that they must be error-free. To reverse this trend, faculty and administration must integrate into their programs the techniques utilized in medical education, which force the medical student to face the limitations of knowledge and of the practitioner.

Structural Changes

Utilization of Feedback within the System   The system needs mechanisms that give a powerful and respected voice to individuals at the bottom of the ladder. Students and floor nurses are seldom listened to. In most institutions, the rating system points downward; administrators rate faculty and faculty members rate students. Supervisors rate staff nurses and nursing administrators rate supervisors. If the students' rating of the faculty and the staff nurses' rating of the supervisors and administration were a respected variable in terms of raises and promotions, some of the authoritarianism within the system might be corrected.

Most schools have exit interviews with students when they complete or leave the program for any reason, and some schools utilize faculty rating scales after each course. However, the administration rarely has to pay attention to the findings. The NLN Monograph on Students' Responsibilities (1977) notes that the Council of Baccalaureate and Higher Degree Programs has consistently acknowledged its concern for students and supported student involvement in the affairs of nursing. This has led to an increasingly active involvement of baccalaureate and graduate students in curriculum development, program evaluation, and the preparation of self-study reports for accreditation purposes. This increasing collaboration between students and faculty has many benefits:

> A fertile area for the identification and nurturing of leaders for nursing; an increase in the quality of the program; a clearer presentation of nursing theory with the concomitant improvement in the operationalization of nursing theory resulting in better health and nursing care for clients; an increase in mutual respect—students for faculty and faculty for students—plus an appreciation for the contribution of both to program development; and an enrichment for the profession of nursing through this mutual sharing of responsibility for education by a community of scholars.*

Despite all these advantages, the pamphlet expresses concern about too much student participation: "Our concern is that what appears to be an overemphasis on student rights may produce an imbalance of knowledge of rights without concomitant knowledge of responsibilities. To recognize and to fullfill one's responsibilities—provided that the appropriate breadth and depth of knowledge has been acquired—is an exercise in thinking and therefore is power." A fear of student power prompted the publication of this pamphlet and permeates its suggestions.

*From The National League of Nursing. 1977. *Students Have Responsibilities As Well As Rights*. Pub. No. 15-1666, p. 2.

Particular concern is expressed about students wanting to participate without attending all the necessary meetings or doing all the necessary reading or homework involved in the task at hand. The pamphlet asserts that students will not have the appropriate breadth and depth of knowledge needed to make important decisions. How could they? Students are still in the process of learning and have not acquired the breadth and depth of knowledge of the educators. As such, this pamphlet provides in liberal terminology a rationale for the fears of all administrators and faculty members: If power is given to students, it will be overemphasized and abused; students do not have the necessary knowledge to make important decisions.

Indeed, they may not have this knowledge. What they can do is give valuable information to the faculty and administrators about what is happening in the institution. My colleagues and I found that students do not utilize faculty rating scales hostilely or carelessly (HEW Grant, 1975). They were quite capable of differentiating between their personal dislikes and the faculty members' abilities and strengths. Many disliked teachers were rated high in terms of teaching ability and knowledge of the subject matter.

Student ratings of faculty should be included in faculty members' evaluations, and supervisors should be evaluated by their subordinates. This does not mean that the student or new graduate will have the only say in matters such as promotion, policy, salary increase, or curriculum; however, their opinions should carry some real weight. Nursing has a long way to go before the rights of students (much less the newly graduated nurse) are overemphasized. If the feedback process is to serve as a corrective, the structure must allow students and beginning nurses a real voice in evaluations.

Integrating the Group Process into the Curriculum   Another structural approach is the utilization of the group processes developed by Kramer (1974) and Cohen and Gesner (1972) and outlined in Chapter 10. Either type of program instituted after the student has gained some familiarity and comfort with the technical skills and knowledge would help students manifest the resistance of Stage II and turn to their peers for support. Both techniques allow students to direct their resistance and questioning into appropriate channels, utilizing the peer group for support and thus facilitating their professional socialization.

Changing the Length of the Educational Process   Two parameters that must be looked at are the age at which students enter school and the length of education. Typically, students begin their nursing education after high school and spend a short period of time on the wards. (Even B.S.N. graduates spend only 2 years on the wards.) Most professions demand longer schooling and a lengthier period of strict supervision. Medical students usually spend 3–4 years as an undergraduate, 4 years as a medical student (including 2 years on wards), and at least 3 years of apprenticeship after graduation.

Nursing programs usually do not expect new graduates to be fully-formed professionals (Stage IV) until 6 months to 2 years after graduation.

However, while there are orientation programs for newly graduated nurses, the programs are not standardized. Most orientation is left to chance or structured according to the needs of the health care institution. A formal extension of the educational period to cover the first year after graduation as an "internship," with supervised clinical experience under real and not overly protected working conditions, would help both the institutions and the new graduate.

Assuming Control of the Professional Data Base and Role Definition Down with the Doctor-Nurse game! This last solution is the most important and the most difficult to implement. Despite Rogers' (1972) contention that the nurse's role is not dictated by another profession, and the repeated efforts of nursing educators to bring professional equality into doctor-nurse interactions (Thomstead, 1975), the game still goes on. Ask any student.

In order to become truly professional, nursing must not only define but have control over its data base. This means not only dealing with its own internal authoritarianism, but conquering the authoritarianism that is present throughout the health field.

How to do this will take investigation of the current field and decisions about areas that nursing can call its own. Altering the educational system to eliminate the enforced dependency and the stifling of resistance (attributes postulated as necessary to the process of becoming professional) will be a long step in the direction of effective socialization.

Conclusion

Grissum (1976) believes nursing's lack of autonomy is caused by the femaleness of the profession. If this is the case, perhaps the women's liberation movement will intercede. If that is too slow, expanding the field to include more males might be a solution. Men would, presumably, demand more power and status. However, both solutions are passive at their core: one awaits a political movement for guidance, the other perpetuates traditional female submissiveness by relying on others to demand freedom and autonomy. (It reminds one of Florence Nightingale, who always found men to speak for her!)

Perhaps my most solid recommendation is to beware of looking to others for the ultimate solution to nursing problems. The solution or solutions must come from within the nursing field. Nurses must actively seek a solution themselves. I can only help conceptualize the problems. Nurses and social scientists share a commitment to education and knowledge. It is hoped that the conceptual framework and data presented here will help nursing educators and administrators put that commitment to work and find solutions to the problems that prevent nursing from becoming truly professional.

NOTES

1. The problem with allowing outside influence on students in the professionalization
   process is a serious one, and nursing educators are justified in their concern. During the course of the HEW project, two therapists were markedly more successful
   than the rest of the staff, both in the numbers of students who sought them out
   and the results of the crisis therapy; the students they treated graduated. One
   therapist was a man in his late twenties, handsome, bearded, "with it," and in the
   process of completing his dissertation. The other was the director, a woman in her
   late thirties who was balancing a career as a clinical psychologist with a home and
   young children.

   When the follow-up data on the crisis program was analyzed 4 years after the students graduated, it became apparent that the female therapist was dangerous to
   nursing education. Nurses who had been counseled by her were leaving nursing
   for other fields—law, social work, and, of course, clinical psychology. Fourteen
   of her cases rated most successful in outcome were in educational programs that
   would remove them from nursing forever. In contrast, the male therapist's 15
   most successful cases were all still very much in nursing. They too had gone on for
   more education, but had remained in nursing—frequently at the same hospital—and were beginning to assume positions of responsibility and power within
   that structure.

   This finding can be explained by the role-model effect. The students were not
   satisfied with the faculty role models. As one said to the female therapist, "Why
   do you have so much more fun than anyone else here?" The ability of the director
   to define her own professional role and her enjoyment of that autonomy contrasted markedly with the nursing faculty. The implicit message to her clients was:
   If you want autonomy, change fields. The male therapist's message was: Go get
   power and then change things.

References

Abdellah, F. 1969. The nature of nursing science. *Nursing Research* 13:388-389.

Adams, J. 1970. Considerations in assesssing changes in personality characteristics of nursing students. *Journal of Psychiatric Nursing* 8(4):12-16.

Adams, J. and Klein, L.R. 1970. Students in nursing school: Consideration in assessing personality characteristics. *Nursing Research* 19:362-366.

Aichlmayer, R.H. 1969. A need to identify and develop the creative student. *Journal of Nursing Education* 18(19):19-27.

Alutto, A., and others. 1971. A study of differential socialization for members of one professional occupation. *Journal of Health and Social Behavior* 12(June):140-147.

American Nurse's Association Committee on Education. 1965. Position on education for nursing. *American Journal of Nursing* 65(Dec.):106.

ANA Convention. 1978. Descriptive write-up. *Nursing Outlook* 26:30-41.

Angrist, S. 1969. The study of sex roles. *Journal of Social Issues* 25(1):215-229.

Armitage, B. 1976. Professional socialization of nurses: A dean's view. *Journal of the New York State Nurses' Association* 4(4):16-20.

Armor, D., and Klerman, G. 1968. Psychiatric treatment orientations and professional ideology. *Journal of Health and Social Behavior* 9(3):228-233.

Ashley, J., and LaBelle, B. 1976. Education for freeing minds. In Williamson, J. (editor): *Current Perspectives in Nursing Education: The changing scene.* St. Louis, Mo.: The C.V. Mosby Co.

Aydelotte, M.K. 1975. Nursing education in practice: Putting it all together. In *Focus on Professional Issues.* Wakefield, Mass.: Contemporary Publishing Co., Inc.

Bailey, J.T., and Claus, K.E. 1969. Comparative analysis of the personality structure of nursing students. *Nursing Research* 18:321-326.

Barnartt, S. 1976. *Sex differences in predictors of attachment to the professional role among medical students.* Ph.D. dissertation, University of Chicago.

Barnartt, S., and Cohen, H.A. 1976. *Becoming a professional: Socialization as an active process.* Unpublished paper. HEW Grant. Chicago: Cook County School of Nursing.

Bates, B. 1975. Doctor and nurse: Changing roles and relations. In *Focus on Professional Issues.* Wakefield, Mass.: Contemporary Publishing Co., Inc.

Batey, M.V. 1969. The two normative worlds of the university nursing faculty. *Nursing Forum* 8(1):5-16.

Bayer, A.E., and Schoenfeldt, L.F. 1970. Student interchangeability in three-year and four-year nursing programs. *The Journal of Human Resources* 5(1):71-88.

Beaver, A. 1953. Personality factors in choice of nursing. *Journal of Applied Psychology* 39:374-379.

Becker, H., and Geer, B. 1961. Latent culture: A note on the theory of latent social roles. *Administrative Science Quarterly* 5:304-313.

Becker, H., and others. 1961. *Boys in White: Student Culture in Medical School.* Chicago: University of Chicago Press.

Benne, K.D., and Bennis, W. 1959(a). The role of the professional nurse. *American Journal of Nursing* 59:196-198.

Benne, K.D., and Bennis, W. 1959(b). What is real nursing? *American Journal of Nursing* 59:380-383.

Benne, K.D., and others. 1975. *The Laboratory Method of Changing and Learning: Theory and Application.* Palo Alto, Calif.: Science and Behavior Books, Inc.

Bennett, G., and Gordon, H. 1944. Personality test scores and success in the field of nursing. *Journal of Applied Psychology* 30:267-278.

Bernard, J. 1964. *Academic Women.* New York: McGraw-Hill Book Co.

Bernstein, L., Turrel, E.S., and Dana, R.H. 1965. Motivation for nursing. *Nursing Research* 15:337-342.

Birnbaum, C. 1975. The C group. In Benne, K.D., and others (editors): *The Laboratory Method of Changing and Learning: Theory and Application.* Palo Alto, Calif.: Science and Behavior Books, Inc.

Bradford, L.P., Gibb, J.R., and Benne, K.D. 1964. *T-Group Theory and Laboratory Method.* New York: John Wiley & Sons.

Brandt, E.M., Hastie, B., and Schumann, D. 1967. Comparison of on-the-job performance of graduates with school of nursing objectives. *Nursing Research* 16:51-60.

Braverman, I.K., and others. 1972. Sex role stereotypes: A current appraisal. *Journal of Social Issues* 29(2):59-78.

Brown, J.S., Swift, Y.B., and Oberman, M.L. 1974. Baccalaureate students' images of nursing: A replication. *Nursing Research* 23:53-59.

Bucher, R. 1970. Social process and power in a medical school. In Zald, M.N. (editor): *Power in Organizations.* Nashville: Vanderbilt University Press.

Bucher, R., and Stelling, J. 1977. Becoming professional. *Sage Library of Social Research,* vol. 46. Beverly Hills: Sage Publications.

Bucher, R., and Strauss, A. 1961. Professions in process. *American Journal of Sociology* 66:325-334.

Bullough, B. 1975(a). Barriers to the nurse practitioner movement: Problems of women in a women's field. *International Journal of Health Services* 5(2):309-317.

Bullough, B. 1975(b). *The Law and the Expanding Nurse Role.* Englewood Cliffs, N.J.: Appleton-Century-Crofts.

Bullough, B., and Bullough, V., editors. 1977. *Expanding Horizons for Nurses.* New York: Springer Publishing Co., Inc.

Bullough, B., and Sparks, C. 1975. Baccalaureate vs. associates degree nurses: The care-cure dichotomy. *Nursing Outlook* 23(11):688-692.

Cambell, D. 1971. *Why Would A Girl Go Into Medicine?* Old Westbury, N.Y.: Feminist Press.

Caplan, G. 1964. *Principles of Preventive Psychiatry.* New York: Basic Books, Inc.

Caplowitz, D. 1961. Student-faculty relations in medical school: A Study of professional socialization. Ph.D. dissertation, Columbia University.

Caputo, V., and Hanf, C. 1965. EPPS patterns and the nursing personality. *Educational and Psychological Measures* 25:421-435.

Casella, C. 1968. Need hierarchies among nursing and nonnursing college students. *Nursing Research* 17:273-275.

Cattell, R.B. 1952. *Factor Analysis.* New York: Harper & Row Publishers.

Christman, L. 1976. Educational standards versus professional performance. In Williamson, J. (editor): *Current Perspectives in Nursing Education: The Changing Scene.* St. Louis: The C.V. Mosby Co.

Christman, J. 1971. Clinical performance of baccalaureate graduates. *Nursing Outlook* 19(1):54-56.

Cleland, V. 1971. Sex discrimination: Nursing's most pervasive problem. *American Journal of Nursing* 71:1542-1547.

Cleveland, S.E. 1961. Personality patterns associated with the dietitian and nurse. *Journal of Health and Human Behavior* 2:113-124.

Cogswell, B.E. 1967. The rehabilitation of the paraplegic: Processes of socialization. *Sociological Inquiry* 37:11-26.

Cohen, E.D., and others. 1974. Women in medicine: Exigencies in training and career. Unpublished paper.

Cohen, H.A. 1976. A Comparison of two consultation training programs. *Professional Psychology* 7(4):533-540.

Cohen, H.A. (principal investigator). 1975. To facilitate learning by providing a multivaried attack on the problem of attrition and staff-student relations. HEW Report 05000309-04 NOD10.

Cohen, H.A. (principal investigator). 1975a. Review of literature section. HEW Report 05000309-04NOO10.

Cohen, H.A., and Gesner, P. 1972. Dropouts and failures: A preventive program. *Nursing Outlook* 20(11):723-725.

Cohen, H.A., and Orlinsky, N. 1977. Work stress on critical care units. *The Journal of Emergency Medical Services* 6(1):31-37.

Conant, L.H. 1967. Closing the practice theory gap. *Nursing Outlook* 15(11):37-39.

Corwin, R.G. 1961. The professional employee: A study of conflict in nursing roles. In Skipper, J.K., and Leonard, R.C. (editors): *Social Interaction and Patient Care.* Philadelphia: J.B. Lippincott Co.

Corwin, R.G., Taves, M., and Haas, J. 1961. Professional disillusionment. *Nursing Research* 10:141-144.

Crichton, M. 1971. *Five Patients.* New York: Bantam Books, Inc.

Crocker, L.M., and Brodie, B.J. 1974. Development of a scale to assess student nurses' views of the professional nursing role. *Journal of Applied Psychology* 59(2):233-235.

Davis, A.J. 1969. Self-concept, occupational role expectation, and occupational choice in nursing and social work. *Nursing Research* 18:55-59.

Davis, F., and Olesen, V.L. 1963. Initiation into a women's profession: Identity problems in the status transition of coed to student nurse. *Sociometry* 26(1):89-101.

Davis, F., and Olesen, V.L. 1964. Baccalaureate students' images of nursing. *Nursing Research* 13:8-15.

Davis, F., and Olesen, V.L. 1965. The career outlook of professionally educated women. *Psychiatry* 28(4):334-345.

Davis, F., Olesen, V.L., and Whittaker, E.W. 1966. Problems and issues in collegiate nursing education. In Davis, F. (editor): *The Nursing Profession: Five Sociological Essays.* New York: John Wiley and Sons, Inc.

De Tornyay, R. 1977. Changing students relationships, roles and responsibilities. *Nursing Outlook* 25(March):188-193.

Dickoff, J., and James, P. 1975. Theory development in nursing. In Verhonick, P.J. (editor): *Nursing Research* 1st ed. Boston: Little, Brown and Co., Inc.

Diers, D. 1976. Nursing: A career for college graduates: A combined basic-graduate program for college graduates. *Nursing Outlook* 24(2):92-98.

Dreeben, R. 1968. The contribution of schooling to the learning of norms. In socialization in the Schools Reprint Series No. 1, *Harvard Educational Review,* pp. 23-49.

Dustan, L.C. 1964. Characteristics of students in three types of nursing education programs. *Nursing Research* 13(2):159-166.

Edwards, A.L. 1969. *Manual for the Edwards Personal Preference Schedule.* New York: Psychological Corp.

Edwards, C.N. 1963. Cultural dissonance and dissimulation: A study in role conflict. *Journal of Consulting and Clinical Psychology* 32:607-610.

Edwards, C.N. 1969. The student nurse: A study in sex role transition. *Psychological Reports* 25:975-990.

Eisenman, R. 1970. Creativity change in student nurses: A cross-sectional and longitudinal study. *Developmental Psychology* 3(3):320-325.

Elms, R.R., and Moorehead, J.M. 1977. Will the "real nurse" please stand up: The stereotype vs. reality. *Nursing Forum* 16(2):112-115.

Epstein, C. 1970. *Woman's Place: Options and Limits in Professional Careers.*Berkeley, Calif.: University of California Press.

Erikson, E. 1950. *Childhood and Society.* New York: W.W. Norton and Co., Inc.

Eron, L.D. 1953. Responses of women to TAT. *Journal of Consulting Psychology* 17:269-282.

Eron, L.D. 1955. The effect of nursing education on attitudes. *Nursing Research* 4:24-27.

Evans, R.I. 1967. *Dialogue with Erik Erikson.* New York: Harper & Row Publishers.

Feldbaum, E. 1977. Integration strategies for the nursing profession, first year report. HEW Division of Nursing, Grant NU0057.

Flint, R.T., and Spensley, K.C. 1969. Recent issues in nursing manpower: A review. *Nursing Research* 18:217-220.

Ford, A. 1950. Prediction of academic success in three schools of nursing. *Journal of Applied Psychology.* 34:186-189.

Fox, R. 1957. Training for uncertainty. In Merton, R., Reader, G., and Kendall, P. (editors): *The Student Physician.* Cambridge, Mass.: Harvard University Press.

French, J. 1961. A predictive test battery. *Nursing Research* 10:104-105.

Friedson, E. 1970. *The Profession of Medicine: A Study in the Sociology of Applied Knowledge.* New York: Dodd, Mead and Co., Inc.

Fromm, L. 1977. The problem in nursing: Nurses! *Supervisor Nurse* 8(Oct.):15-16.

Gerstein, A. 1965. Development of a selection program for nursing candidates. *Nursing Research* 14:254-275.

Getzels, J.W., and Jackson, P.W. 1962. *Creativity and Intelligence.* New York: John Wiley and Sons.

Ginzburg, E. 1966. *Life Styles of Educated Women.* New York: Columbia University Press.

Goffman, E. 1959. *The Presentation of Self in Every Day Life.* New York: Anchor Books.

Goffman, E. 1961(a). *Asylums.* New York: Anchor Books.

Goffman, E. 1961(b). Role distance. In *Encounters.* New York: Bobbs-Merrill Co., Inc.

Goode, W.J. 1972. Community within a community: The professions. In Pavalko, R.M. (editor): *Sociological Perspectives on Occupations.* Itasca, Ill.: F.E. Peacock Publishers, Inc.

Gortner, S.R. 1968. Nursing majors in twelve western universities: A comparison of registered nurse students and basic senior students. *Nursing Research* 17:121-128.

Gouldner, F. 1957. Cosmopolitans and locals: Toward an analysis of latent social roles.

Administrative Science Quarterly 2:281-306.

Grandjean, B.D., Aiken, L.H., and Bonjean, C.M. 1976. Professional autonomy and the work satisfaction of nursing educators. *Nursing Research* 25:216-221.

Greenwood, E. 1972. Attributes of a profession. In Pavalko, R. (editor): *Sociological Perspectives on Occupations.* Itasca, Ill.: F.E. Peacock Publishers, Inc.

Grissum, M., and Spengler, C. 1976. *Womanpower and Health Care.* Boston: Little, Brown and Co., Inc.

Group, T.M., and Roberts, J.I. 1974. Exorcising the ghosts of the Crimea. *Nursing Outlook* 22(6):368-372.

Guilford, J.P. 1967. *The Nature of Human Intelligence.* New York: McGraw-Hill Book Co.

Gunter, L.M. 1969. The developing nursing student (part II): Attitudes toward nursing as a career. *Nursing Research* 18:131-136.

Habenstein, R., and Christ, E. 1955. *Professionalizer, Traditionalizer, and Utilizer.* Columbia, Mo.: University of Missouri Press.

Hadley, B.J. 1969. Evolution of a conception of nursing. *Nursing Research* 18:400-405.

Hall, O. 1948. The stages of a medical career. *American Journal of Sociology* 53(2):327-336.

Handlin, O. 1952. *The Uprooted.* Boston: Little, Brown and Co., Inc.

Harvey, L.H. 1970. Educational problems of minority group nurses. *Nursing Outlook* 18(9):48-50.

Harvey, O.J., Hunt, D.E., and Schroder, H.M. 1961. *Conceptual Systems and Personality Organization.* New York: John Wiley and Sons, Inc.

Hassenplug, L.W. 1977. Nursing can move from here to there. *Nursing Outlook* 10(4):432-438.

HEW Report No. 05000309-04 NOD10. 1975. To facilitate learning by providing a multi-varied attack on the problem of attrition and staff-student relations. Cohen, H.A., Ph.D., principal investigator.

Henry, W.E., and Sims, J.E. 1970. Actions in search for a self. *Trans-action* Sept.:57-62.

Highrighter, M.D. 1969. Nursing characteristics and patient progress. *Nursing Research* 18(3):4848-500.

Hillsmith, K. 1978. From RN to BSN: Student perceptions. *Journal of Advanced Nursing* 3:369-372.

Horner, M. 1969. Fail: Bright women. *Psychology Today* (November).

Hott, J.R. 1977. Updating Cherry Ames. *American Journal of Nursing* 77:1581-1583.

Hover, J. 1975. Diploma vs. degree nurses: Are they alike? *Nursing Outlook* 23(11):684-687.

Howard, K.I., and Gordon, R.A. 1963. Empirical note on the "number of factors" problem in factor analysis. *Psychological Reports* 12:247-250.

Hughes, E.C., Hughes, H., and Deutscher, I. 1958. *Twenty Thousand Nurses Tell Their Story.* Philadelphia: J.B. Lippincott Co.

Hutcheson, J.D., Garland, L.M., and Prather, J.E. 1973. Toward reducing attrition in baccalaureate degree nursing programs: An exploratory study. *Nursing Research* 22:530-533.

Ingmire, A.E. 1952. Attitudes of student nurses at the University of California. *Nursing Research* 1:36-39.

Inkles, A. 1968. The social structure and socialization of competence. In socialization in the Schools Reprints Series No. 1, *Harvard Educational Review,* pp. 50-68.

Israel, J., and Sjorstrand, P. 1968. Generalized role as a factor influencing the learning of professional values and attitudes. *Acta Sociolǫgica* 11:177-192.

Jacox, A. 1973. Professional socialization of nurses. *Journal of the New York State Nurses' Association* 4(4):6-15.

Jacox, A. 1978. Progress to the next generation. *Nursing Outlook* 26:38-41.

Johnson, D. 1966. Competence in practice: Technical and professional. *Nursing Outlook* 10(Oct.):30-33.

Johnson, M., and Martin, H.W. 1958. A sociological analysis of the nurse role. *American Journal of Sociology* 58(Mar.):373-377.

Johnson, R.W., and Leonard, L.C. 1970. Psychological test characteristics and performance of nursing students. *Nursing Research* 19:147-150.

Jones, S.L. 1976. Socialization versus selection factors as source of student definitions of the nurse role. *Journal of Nursing Studies* 13:135-138.

Kaplan, H. 1970. Women physicians: The more effective recruitment and utilization of their talents and the resistance to it — the final conclusions of a seven-year study. *The Woman Physician* 25:561-571.

Katz, F.E. 1969. Nurses. In Etzioni, A. (editor): *The Semi-Professions and Their Organization.* New York: The Free Press.

Katz, F.E., and Martin, M.W. 1972. Career choice processes. In Pavalko, R.M. (editor): *Sociological Perspectives on Occupations.* Itasca, Ill.: F.E. Peacock Publishers.

Katzell, M.E. 1968. Expectations and dropouts in schools of nursing. *Journal of Applied Psychology* 52(2):154-157.

Kelly, W.L. 1974. Psychological predictions of leadership in nursing. *Nursing Research* 23:38-42.

Kelman, H. 1967. Three processes of social influence. In *Current Perspectives in Social Psychology.* New York: Oxford University Press.

Khlief, B. 1974. Professionalization of psychiatric residents. In Steward, E., and Cantor, J., (editors): *Variations of Work Experience.* New York: John Wiley and Sons, Inc.

Kibrick, A.K. 1963. Dropouts in schools of nursing. *Nursing Research* 12:140-149.

Kibrick, A.K., and Tiedeman, D.V., 1961. Conceptions of self and perception of role in schools of nursing. *Journal of Counseling Psychology* 8(1):62-69.

King, I.M. 1975. A Process for developing concepts for nursing through research. In Verhonick, P.J. (editor): *Nursing Research* 1st ed. Boston: Little, Brown and Co., Inc.

Klett, C.J. 1957. Performance of high school students on the Edwards Personal Preference Schedule. *Journal of Consulting Psychology* 21:68-72.

Knopf, L. 1975. *Graduation and Withdrawal from R.N. Programs.* U.S. Department of Health, Education, and Welfare. Pub. No. 19-1535.

Kohnke, M.F. 1973. Do nursing educators practice what is preached? *American Journal of Nursing* 73:1571-1578.

Kramer, M. 1968. Role models, role conceptions, and role deprivation. *Nursing Research* 17:115-120.

Kramer, M. 1969. Collegiate graduate nurses in medical center hospitals: Mutual challenge or duel? *Nursing Research* 18:196-210.

Kramer, M. 1974. *Reality Shock: Why Nurses Leave Nursing.* St. Louis: The C.V. Mosby Co.

Krueger, C. 1968. Do "bad girls" become good nurses? *Trans-action* 5(July/Aug.):31-36.

Lambertsen, E.C. 1953. *Nursing Team Organization and Functioning.* Cited in Meyer, G.R. 1959. Conflict and harmony in nursing values. *Nursing Outlook* 7(July):398-399.

Lambertsen, E.C. 1975. Let's get the nurse's role into perspective. In *Focus on Professional Issues.* Wakefield, Mass.: Contemporary Publishing Co., Inc.

Leininger, M. 1969. The nature of science in nursing. *Nursing Research* 18:388-389.

Leonard, R.C., and others. 1975. Etiology and control of stress in clinical settings. In Verhonick, P.J. (editor): *Nursing Research* 1st ed. Boston: Little, Brown and Co., Inc.

Leventhal, H., and Israel, S. 1975. The behavioral measure: Conceptualizing, researching and analyzing the psychological factors in nursing research. In Verhonick,

P.J. (editor): *Nursing Research* 1st ed. Boston: Little, Brown and Co., Inc.

Levitt, E.E., Lubin, B., and Zuckerman, M. 1962. The student nurse, the college woman, and the graduate nurse: A Comparative study. *Nursing Research* 11:80-82.

Lewis, F.M. 1976. The nurse as lackey: A sociological perspective. *Supervisor Nurse* 7(April):24-27.

Lieberman, M.A., Yalom, I.D., and Miles, M.B. 1971. The group experience project: A comparison of ten encounter technologies. In Blank, L., Gottsegen, G.B., and Gottsegen, M.G. (editors): *Encounter: Confrontations in Self and Interpersonal Awareness.* New York: Macmillan Publishing Co.

Lief, H., and Fox, R. 1963. The medical student's training for detached concern, in Lief, V., Lief, H., and Lief, F. (editors): *The Psychological Basis of Medical Practice.* New York: Harper & Row Publishers.

Lysaught, J.P., editor. 1971. *Abstract For Action.* McGraw-Hill Book Co.

Lysaught, J.P., editor. 1973. *Abstract Into Action.* McGraw-Hill Book Co.

Malher, D. 1955. Use of MMPI with student nurses. *Journal of Applied Psychology* 39:190-193.

Mauksch, H.O. 1963. Becoming a nurse: A selective view. *Annals of the American Academy of Social and Political Sciences* 346:88-98.

Mauksch, H.O. 1972. Nursing: Churning for change? In Freeman, F., and others (editors): *Handbook of Medical Sociology* 2nd ed. Beverly Hills: Sage Press.

Mauksch, I.G. 1975. Attaining control over professional practice. In *Focus on Professional Issues.* Wakefield, Mass.: Contemporary Publishing Co., Inc.

May, W.T. 1966. Differences between nursing student drop-outs and remainers on study of values. *Psychological Reports* 3(1):902.

May, W.T., and Ilardi, R.L. 1970. Image and stability of values of collegiate nursing students. *Nursing Research* 19:359-361.

McCall, G., and Simmons, J. 1966. *Identities and Interactions.* New York: The Free Press.

McDonald, T.D., and others. 1969. Occupational choice, commitment, values, and orientations of nursing students. *Indian Sociological Bulletin* 7(1):1-11.

McKay, R. 1969. Theories, models and systems for nursing. *Nursing Research* 18:393-399.

McKee, J.B. 1969. *Introduction to Sociology.* New York: Holt, Rinehart & Winston, Inc.

Meleis, A.I., and Farrell, K.M. 1974. Operation concern: A study of senior nursing students in three nursing programs. *Nursing Research* 23:461-468.

Merrill, R., and Murphy, D. 1965. Predicting academic success for nursing students. *Nursing Research* 14:341-344.

Merton, R., Reader, G., and Kendall, P. 1957. *The Student Physician: Introductory Studies in the Sociology of Medical Education.* Cambridge, Mass.: Harvard University Press.

Merton, R.K. 1968. *Social Theory and Social Structure.* New York: The Free Press.

Meyer, G.R. 1959. Conflict and harmony in nursing values. *Nursing Outlook* 7(July): 398-399.

Meyer, G.R. 1960. *Tenderness and Technique: Nursing Values in Transition.* Institute for Industrial Relations. Berkeley, Calif.: University of California.

Michael, J.J., and others. 1971. The criterion related validities of cognitive and noncognitive predictors in a training program for nursing candidates. *Education and Psychological Measurement* 31:983-987.

Miller, M. 1977. Academic inbreeding in nursing. *Nursing Outlook* 25(3):172-177.

Miller, S.M. 1972. The making of a confused, middle-aged husband. In Safilios-Rothschild, C. (editor): *Toward a Sociology of Women.* Lexington, Mass.: Xerox Corp.

Mitchell, R. 1977. *Personal empathy status and professional empathy attribution of nursing students.* Master's dissertation, Illinois Institute of Technology.

Montag, M. 1951. *Education of Nursing Technicians.* New York: G.P. Putnam's Sons.

Montag, M. 1964. The logic of associate degree programs in nursing. *Nursing Science* 2(June):188-197.

Moody, M. 1973. Attitudes of cynicism and humanitarianism in nursing students and staff nurses. *Journal of Nursing Education* 12(Aug.):9-13.

Moore, M.A. 1969. The professional practice of nursing. *Nursing Forum* 18(4):361-373.

Moore, W. 1961. Occupational socialization. In Goslin, D. (editor): *Handbook of Socialization Theory and Research.* New York: Rand McNally & Co.

Munday, L., and Hoyt, D. 1965. Predicting success for nursing students. *Nursing Research* 14:341-344.

National League of Nursing. 1977. *Students Have Responsibilities as Well as Rights.* NLN Pub. No. 15-1666. New York.

National League of Nursing. 1979. *Perspectives for Nursing and Goals of the National League for Nursing 1979-1981.* Pub. No. 11-1782. New York.

Navran, L., and Stauffacher, J.C. 1957. Personality structure of psychiatric nurses. *Nursing Research* 7:125-132.

Neugarten, B. 1946. Social class and friendship among school children. *American Journal of Sociology* 51:305-313.

Newcomb, D.P. 1953. *The Team Plan: A Manual for Nursing Service Administrators.* New York: G.P. Putnam's Sons.

Notter, L., and Spalding, E. 1976. *Professional Nursing: Foundations, Perspectives and Relationships* 9th ed. Philadelphia: J.B. Lippincott Co.

Olesen, V.L. 1973. What happens after schooling. *Social Science and Medicine* 7:61-75.

Olesen, V.L., and Davis, F. 1966. Baccalaureate students' images of nursing: A follow-up report. *Nursing Research* 15:151-158.

Olesen, V.L. and Whittaker, E. 1968. *The Silent Dialogue.* San Francisco: Jossey-Bass, Inc.

Olmsted, G., and Paget, M.A. 1962. Some theoretical issues in professional socialization. *Journal of Medical Education.* 44(8):663-669.

O'Mahoney, M.T., and Cohen, H.A. 1974. *A Typological analysis of personality and attitudinal profiles of student nurses.* Unpublished paper. HEW Grant. Chicago: Cook County School of Nursing.

O'Mahoney, M., and Labbie, S. 1973. Factors of the image of nursing scale and their relation to personality dimensions and GPA. Paper presented at the American Psychological Association Annual Meeting, Montreal.

O'Neill, M.F. 1973. A Study of baccalaureate nursing student values. *Nursing Research* 22:437-443.

Owen, S.V., Feldhusen, J.F., and Thurston, J.R. 1970. Achievement prediction in nursing education with cognitive, attitudinal, and divergent thinking variables. *Psychological Reports* 26:867-870.

Ozimek, D., and Yura, H. 1977. *Students Have Responsibilities As Well As Rights.* National League of Nursing Pub. No. 15-1666. New York.

Pavalko, R. 1971. *Sociology of Occupations and Professions.* Itasca, Ill.: F.E. Peacock Publishers.

Pavalko, R. 1972. *Sociological Perspectives on Occupations.* Itasca, Ill.: F.E. Peacock Publishers.

Pechiulis, D. 1972. The academic honeymoon is over. *Nursing Outlook* 20(3):180-181.

Piaget, J. 1928. *Judgment and Reasoning in the Child.* New York: Harcourt Brace Jovanovich, Inc.

Plapp, J.M., Psathas, G., and Caputo, D.V. 1966. *Effects of Nurse's Training on Personality.* Proceedings of the 74th Annual Convention of the American Psychological Association, 287-288.

Plummer, E.M., and Phelan, M.J. 1976. College graduates in nursing: A retrospective look. *Nursing Outlook* 24(2):99-103.

Psathas, G. 1968. *The Student Nurse in the Diploma School of Nursing.* New York: Springer Publishing Co., Inc.

Psathas, G. 1969. The fate of idealism in nursing schools. *Journal of Health and Social Behavior* 9:52-64.

Quarantelli, E.L., Helfrich, M., and Yutsy, D. 1964. Faculty and student perceptions in a professional school. *Sociology and Social Research* 49(1):32-45.

Quint, J. 1967. Role models and the professional nurse identity. *Journal of Nursing Education* 6(2):11-15.

Raderman, R., and Allen, D.V. 1974. Registered nurse students in a baccalaureate program: Factors associated with completion. *Nursing Resarch* 23:71-73.

Redden, J.W., and Scales, E.E. 1961. Nursing education and personality characteristics. *Nursing Research* 10:215-218.

Reece, M.M. 1961. Personality characteristics and success in a nursing program. *Nursing Research* 10:172-176.

Reed, C.L., Feldhusen, J.F., and Van Mondfrans, A.P. 1972. Prediction of grade point averages in nursing schools using second-order multiple regression models. *Journal of Educational Measurement* 9(3):181-187.

Reed, C.L., Feldhusen, J.F., and Van Mondfrans, A.P. 1973. Prediction of grade point averages using cognitive and noncognitive predictor variables. *Psychological Reports* 32(1):143-148.

Reichow, R.W., and Scott, R.E. 1976. Study compares graduates of two-, three-, and four-year programs. *Hospitals* 50:95-100.

Rein, I. 1977. Medical and nursing students: Concepts of self and ideal self, typical and ideal work partner. *Journal of Personality Assesssment* 41(4):368-374.

Reinkemeyer, A.M. 1968. It won't be hospital nursing. *American Journal of Nursing.* Sept.: 1936-1940.

Reuschmeyer, D. 1972. Doctors and lawyers: A comment on the theory of professions. In Friedson, E., and Lorber, J. (editors): *Medical Men and Their Work.* Chicago: Aldine Publishing Co.

Richards, M.A. 1972. A study of differences in psychological characteristics of students graduating from three types of basic nursing programs. *Nursing Research* 21:259-261.

Richards, R.E. 1978. The game professionals play. *Supervisor Nurse* 6(June):48-50.

Richman, M., and O'Donnell, K. 1978. *The Shikse's Guide to Jewish Men.* New York: Bantam Books, Inc.

Rogers, M.E. 1970. *An Introduction to the Theoretical Basis of Nursing.* Philadelphia: F.A. Davis Co.

Rogers, M.E. 1972. Nursing: To be or not to be. *Nursing Outlook* 20(12):42-46.

Rogoff, N. 1957. The decision to study medicine. In Merton, R., Reader, G., and Kendall, P. (editors): *The Student Physician.* Cambridge, Mass.: Harvard University Press.

Rosen, R.A. 1973. Occupational role innovators and sex role attitudes. *Journal of Medical Education* 49:554-561.

Roth, R. 1970. Underachieving students and guidance. *Guidance and the Exceptional Student.* Guidance Monograph Series V. New York: Houghton Mifflin Co.

Roth, R., and Meyersburg, H. 1963. The nonachievement syndrome. *Personnel and Guidance Journal* 41:535-540.

Roth, R., and Puri, P. 1967. Direction of aggression and the nonachievement syndrome. *Journal of Counseling Psychology* 14:277-281.

Roy, C. 1971. Adaptation: Basis for nursing practice. *Nursing Outlook* 19:254-257.

Saffer, J.B., and Saffer, L.D. 1972. Academic record as a predictor of future job performance of nurses. *Nursing Research* 21:457-462.

Santo, S. 1978. A beginning nurse reacts. *American Journal of Nursing* 78(June):1032-1034.

Schaefer, M.J. 1975. Towards a full profession of nursing: The challenge of the educator's role. In *Focus on Professional Issues*. Wakefield, Mass.: Contemporary Publishing Co., Inc.

Schlotfeldt, R.M. 1975. The need for a conceptual framework. In Verhonick, P.J. (editor): *Nursing Research* 1st ed. Boston: Little, Brown and Co.

Schmidt, M.H. 1968. Role conflict in nursing. *American Journal of Nursing* 68:2348-2350.

Schoeberle, E.A., and Craddick, R.A. 1968. Human figure drawings by freshman and senior student nurses. *Perceptual and Motor Skills* 27:11-14.

Schoenmaker, S., and Radosevich, D. 1976. Men nursing students: How they perceive their situation. *Nursing Outlook* 24(5):298-302.

Schulman, S. 1958. Basic functional roles in nursing: Mother surrogate and healer. In Jaco, E.G. (editor): *Patients, Physicians and Illness*. New York: The Free Press.

Schulman, S. 1972. Mother surrogate — after a decade. In Jaco, E.G. (editor): *Patients, Physicians and Illness* 2nd ed. New York: The Free Press.

Schulz, E.D. 1965. Personality traits of nursing students and faculty concepts of desirable traits: A longitudinal comparative study. *Nursing Research* 14:261-264.

Segal, B.E. 1962. Male nurses: A case study in status contradiction and prestige loss. *Social Forces* 41(1):31-38.

Sharp, W.H., and Anderson, J.C. 1972. Changes in nursing students' descriptions of the personality traits of the ideal nurse. *Measurement and Evaluation in Guidance* 5:339-444.

Sheehy, G. 1974. *Passages*. New York: E.P. Dutton & Co., Inc.

Shaw, M.C., and McCuen, J.T. 1960. The onset of academic underachievement in bright children. *Journal of Educational Psychology* 51:103-108.

Sherlock, B.J., and Morris, R.T. 1967. The evolution of the professional: A Paradigm. *Sociological Inquiry* 37(1):27-46.

Siegel, H. 1968. Professional socialization in two baccalaureate programs. *Nursing Research* 17:403-407.

Simmons, L. 1964. Cited in Schmitt, M. 1968. Role conflict. *American Journal of Nursing* 68(11):00-00.

Simms, S. 1977. Nursing's dilemma — the battle for role determination. *Supervisor Nurse* 8(Sept.):29-31.

Simpson, I.H. 1967. A study of socialization into professions: The case of student nurses. *Sociological Inquiry* 37(1):47-54.

Simpson, R.L., and Simpson, I.H. 1969. Women and bureaucracy in the semiprofessions. In Etzioni, A. (editor): *The Semi-Professions and Their Organizations*. New York: The Free Press.

Smith, J.E. 1968. Personality structure in beginning nursing students: A factor analytic study. *Nursing Research* 17:140-145.

Smith, R.A. 1976. Nursing: A Career for college graduates: Why college graduates choose nursing. *Nursing Outlook* 24(2):88-91.

Smoyak, S. 1969. Toward understanding nursing situations: A transaction paradigm. *Nursing Research* 18(5):405-411.

Sobol, E. 1978. Self-actualization and the baccalaureate nursing student's response to stress. *Nursing Research* 27:238-244.

Solomon, L.N., and Berzon, B., editors. 1972. *New Perspectives on Encounter Groups*. San Francisco: Jossey-Bass, Inc.

Spaney, E. 1953. Personality tests and the selection of nurses. *Nursing Research*. 1:4-26.

Stauffacher, J.C., and Navran, L. 1968. The prediction of subsequent professional
      activity on nursing students by the Edwards Personal Preference Schedule. *Nurs-
      ing Research* 17:256-260.
Stein, L.L. 1971. The doctor-nurse game. In Bullough, B., and Bullough, V. (editors):
      New Directions for Nurses. New York: Springer Publishing Co., Inc.
Stein, R.F. 1969. The student nurse: A study of needs, roles and conflicts (part I).
      Nursing Research 18:308-315.
Stewart, R., and Liggle, J. 1975. Where success lies. *New Zealand Nursing Journal*
      68(3):13-14.
Stone, L.J., editor. 1973. *The Competent Infant: Research and Commentary.* New
      York: Basic Books, Inc.
Stromberg, F.M. 1976. Relationship of sex role identity to occupational image of
      female nursing students. *Nursing Research* 25:363-369.
Stryker, S. 1968. Identity salience and role performance. The relevance of symbolic
      interaction theory for family research. *Journal of Marriage and the Family*
      30(4):558-564.
Sullivan, H.S. 1953. *The Interpersonal Theory of Psychiatry.* New York: W.W. Norton
      and Co., Inc.
Sullivan, J. 1978. Comparison of manifest needs of nurses and physicians in primary
      care practice. *Nursing Research* 27:255-259.
Tate, B. 1961. *Study of Attrition Rates in Schools of Nursing.* New York: National
      League for Nursing, Inc.
Taylor, C., and others. 1966. *Selection and Recruitment of Nurses and Nursing Educa-
      tion: A Review of Research Studies and Practices.* Salt Lake City, Utah: Univer-
      sity of Utah Press.
Teal, G., and Fabrizio, R. 1961. *Causes of Student Withdrawal from Nurses Training.*
      Stamford, Conn.: Public Service Research, Inc.
Tetreault, A.I. 1976. Selected factors associated with professional attitudes of baccalau-
      reate nursing students. *Nursing Research* 25:49-53.
Thomstad, B., and others. 1975. Changing the rules of the doctor-nurse game. *Nursing
      Outlook* 23:(7):422-427.
Thurston, J.R., Brunclik, H.L., and Feldhusen, J.F. 1969. Personality and the predic-
      tion of success in nursing. *Nursing Research* 18:258-262.
Torrance, P.N. 1964. Does nursing education reduce creativity? *Nursing Outlook*
      July:27-30.
Travisano, R. 1970. Alternation and conversion as qualitatively different transforma-
      tions. In Stone, G., and Farberman, H. (editors): *Sociology through Symbolic
      Interaction Theory.* Waltham, Mass.: Ginn-Blaisdell.
Ventura, M. 1976. Related social behaviors of students in different types of nursing edu-
      cation programs. *International Journal of Nursing Studies* 13:3-10.
Ventura, M.R., and Meyers, C.R. 1976. Creative thinking abilities of student nurses.
      Psychological Reports 39:409-410.
Wagner, P. 1976. The Roy adaptation model: Testing the adaptation model in practice.
      Nursing Outlook 24:682-685.
Wang, R., and Watson, J. 1977. The professional nurse: Roles, competencies and char-
      acteristics. *Supervisor Nurse* 8(June):69-71.
Warnecke, R.B. 1973. Nonintellectual factors related attrition from a collegiate nursing
      program. *Journal of Health and Social Behavior* 14(June):153-166.
Watson, J. 1977. Role conflict in nursing. *Supervisor Nurse* 8(July):50.
Watson, J. 1978. Conceptual systems of undergraduate nursing students as compared
      with university students at large and practicing nurses. *Nursing Research* 27:151-155.
Wells, H. 1944. *Cherry Ames, Senior Nurse.* New York: Grosset and Dunlap, Inc.

Werner, M.A. 1973. Professional socialization of nurses: A faculty member's view. *Journal of the New York State Nurses' Association* 4(4):23-25.

Wersgerber, C.A. 1951. Predictive value of MMPI and student nurses. *Journal of Social Psychology* 33:3-11.

Wersgerber, C.A. 1954. Norms for MMPI with student nurses. *Journal of Clinical Psychology* 10:192-194.

Williams, D. 1976. An analysis of nursing state board scores according to Myer-Briggs personality types. *Dissertation Abstracts* 36(8A):5167.

Williams, M., Bloch, D., and Blair, E. 1978. Values and value changes of graduate nursing students: Their relationship to faculty values and selected educational factors. *Nursing Research* 27:181-189.

Williams, T.R., and Williams, M.M. 1959. The socialization of the student nurse. *Nursing Research* 8:18-25.

Williamson, J.A. 1972. The conflict-producing role of the professionally socialized nurse-faculty member. *Nursing Forum* 11(4):356-366.

Williamson, J., editor. 1976. *Current Perspective in Nursing Education: The Changing Scene.* St. Louis: The C.V. Mosby Co.

Willman, M. 1976. Changes in nursing students. In Williamson, J. (editor): *Current Perspectives in Nursing Education: The Changing Scene.* St. Louis: The C.V. Mosby Co.

Wilson, H., and Levy, J. 1978. Why R.N. students drop out. *Nursing Outlook* 26:437-441.

Wilson, V. 1971. An analysis of femininity in nursing. *American Behavioral Scientist* 15(2):213-220.

Winstead-Fry, P. 1977. The need to differentiate a nursing self. *American Journal of Nursing* Sept. 77:1452-1454.

Wood, L. 1973. Proposal: A career plan for nursing. *American Journal of Nursing* 73(5):832-835.

Woolley, A. 1978. From R.N. to B.S.N.: Faculty perceptions. *Journal of Advanced Nursing* 3(July):373-379.

Wren, G. 1971. Some characteristics of freshman students in baccalaureate, diploma, and associate degree nursing programs. *Nursing Research* 20:167-172.

Zucher, L.A. 1967. Learning the seaman role in a total institution. *Sociological Inquiry* 37(1):28-98.

APPENDICES

Appendix A

THE PROFESSIONAL SOCIALIZATION PROCESS IN MEDICAL EDUCATION

Medical schools are especially efficient in pushing their students through the cognitive stages. Their low dropout rate (4% males, 8% females; Kaplan, 1970) is partly a result of a rigorous selection process and partly a result of the educational structures and social climate. What structures and social climate in medical school help students attain their goal, even though it is a long and sometimes tedious journey?

Structure   Although curricula vary, certain basic features are universal. During the preclinical years, students are taught in large groups. Primarily, time is spent in lectures and labs, and students commonly complain that they are overwhelmed by the amount of work required. Generally, the basic science courses are taught to large classes in the preclinical period by science faculty Ph.D.s rather than by M.D.s. Since the basic science faculty members are not practitioners, they sometimes teach material that students (Becker and others, 1961) and medical faculty (Bucher, 1970) consider inappropriate. Large classes preclude questioning of the professors, but interaction among students produces a student culture. This student culture encourages studying to pass exams and simply getting through the material, not learning for future use (Becker and others, 1961).

Subsequently, the apprenticeship experience starts. Students rotate in small groups through basic clerkships in a clinical setting. Contacts are primarily with house staff, attending physicians, and patients. The same small group of peers progresses through training together.

During their apprenticeship, medical students begin to assume the role of physician. The rapid fire give-and-take format of rounds (Crichton, 1971) encourages quick application of theory to practice. Students take medical histories, do physical examinations, make diagnoses, and prescribe treatments. While they cannot prescribe drugs, they can suggest types of treatment. These are the tasks they will practice as professionals, except that as students they are not legally responsible for their decisions.

CULTURAL CLIMATE

Two aspects of the cultural climate in medical school are important in the socialization of medical students. The very high status of physicians in our society affects the process, as does the manner in which instructors teach neophytes how to deal with the problems of life and death — the basis of the professional data base.

On the first point, learning to be a physician becomes a very important part of one's self-concept and a bolster to one's self-esteem. Our society permits subordinating all other relevant roles to the professional identity. The higher the status of the profession, the more this process of subordinating all other relevant roles will be allowed. For example, a busy male physician who sees his children only when they are asleep can still maintain his perception of himself as a good father. Being a good physician means, by definition, that he is a good father — all must understand that professional time comes first. Because of the high status of the physician role, the neophyte is willing to put up with much inconvenience to reach that status. This undoubtedly is a factor in medical schools' low attrition rate.

Equally important in the medical socialization process is the cultural climate, which prepares the physician to deal with the uncertainties of medicine and the gaps and contradictions in its knowledge base. As Fox (1957) states:

> Two basic types of uncertainty may be recognized. The first results from incomplete or imperfect mastery of available knowledge. No one can have at his command all skills and all knowledge of the lore of medicine. The second depends upon limitations of current medical knowledge. There are innumerable questions for which no physician, however knowledgeable, can provide answers. A third source of uncertainty derives from the first two. This consists of difficulty in distinguishing between personal ignorance or ineptitude and the limitations of present medical knowledge.*

An examination of the cognitive stages in medical education will demonstrate the role of uncertainty in medical students' socialization.

*From Fox, R. 1957. Training for uncertainty. In Merton, R., Reader, G., and Kendall, P. (editors): *The Student Physician,* p. 208.

MEDICAL EDUCATION
AND THE COGNITIVE STAGES

When medical students enter the dependent stage, they have already earned an undergraduate premedical degree and learned a great deal of biology. Dependence upon the faculty, however, is insured by frequent examinations based upon copious amounts of memorized material. The students may not feel any particular trust in the instructors since they are usually Ph.D.s and not M.D.s and thus cannot serve as role models, but there is a great deal of inducement for Kelman's (1967) concept of compliance. All the instructors give grades, and although most students know that they probably will not flunk out, there is nevertheless a great deal of competition; the type of internship or residency for which the student will be able to apply depends on his or her grades. It is therefore in the student's best interests to comply with the demands and to depend on the instructors.

Large classes prevent questioning of the professors and insure that students will simply accept the knowledge as presented. However, although large classes preclude questioning, they encourage the interaction among students that produces a student culture. This student culture is based upon resistance. An example of this is what Becker and others (1961) found when they observed that students were studying simply to pass examinations and get through, not to learn the material for later use. This resistance receives covert reinforcement from the medical school staff, which views much of this early material as unnecessary for the practice of medicine (Bucher, 1970).

The climate for the second stage of negative/independence has been set by the time the student begins the clinical clerkship, the apprenticeship experience. Medical students are encouraged to enter Stage II, negative/independence. They are exposed to a variety of role models and can pick and choose those with whom to identify and trust. Autonomy and initiative are demanded. The student who suggests an unusual diagnosis that turns out to be correct is the one whose clinical ability is praised.

The emphasis on the student as chooser and producer of relevant facts may in some schools be in marked contrast to the preclinical emphasis on repeating facts. If the transition from the essentially passive student role to the active apprentice physician role is too fast and abrupt, students may feel overwhelmed. It is here that the groups formed during the first 2 years become helpful. Although time pressures and the large amount of material to be learned may prohibit any formal expression of the resistance of Stage II in the classroom, the result of this time pressure is that students study in groups. (Barnartt [1976] found that most medical students received help from other students or studied with them on a weekly basis.) These study groups pave the way for the clerkship groups that form when the students enter their clinical experience. Just as groups once provided support in learning overwhelming masses of material, they now provide emotional support in dealing with the demands of the clinical experience.

During the preclinical years, the student tends to view all problems with cases as due to his or her own knowledge limitations. This is the dependent approach of Stage I, in which the student tries to learn everything possible and takes information on faith. In the apprenticeship, however, the information cannot be presented in neat packages, and the faculty will make the student conscious of the vastness of medicine's data base. They will convey to him or her, directly or by inference, that even mature physicians do not always know all there is to know. "There are so many voids in medical knowledge, the practice of medicine is sometimes largely a matter of conjuring possibilities and probabilities" (Wells, quoted in Fox, 1957).

The student then turns to peers for support and help in differentiating between two kinds of uncertainty: one's own problems with knowledge and the problems of the field. Through the process of using each other as sounding boards, students learn that uncertainty is experienced by all. By casually joking about this, they begin to set standards for dealing with it. Since faculty members share the experience of limited medical knowledge and guide students to learn in those areas in which knowledge is limited, the faculty become ex officio group members. Faculty members teach students to differentiate between the two kinds of uncertainty. Standards that eventually emerge for dealing with uncertainty coincide with those of the faculty because they have been shaped by faculty participation. Students are permitted a long period in which to adjust to both personal and the field's uncertainties.

Just as the seeds for Stage II, resistance, are inherent in the structures of Stage I, so are the seeds of Stage III, mutuality—in which the student identifies with the peer group and with the other members of the profession and tries on the new role on a protected basis—set in the resistance of Stage II.

Medical education keeps students in Stage III, mutuality, for a long period of time. This is a useful stage for them. The students are exposed to many role models over long periods of time. Upon graduation they are not expected to be full-fledged practitioners, but will go on to internships and residencies. Students at this stage have opportunities to compare notes and to evaluate staff, interns, and residents (Caplowitz, 1961). They can decide who they wish to emulate and try out their own role enactments of the physician's role with peers and supervisors. Not only their bedside manner, but all presentations of self and views of patients and health care will be tried on for size during this time.

Whatever problems students may have with Stage I, dependence, or with Stage II, resistance, appear to be made up for in Stage III, mutuality. Stage III provides a socialization experience that produces a Stage IV independent professional who has a firm identification with the field.

Stage IV (interdependence), in which the neophyte internalizes a manner of presenting the professional role acceptable to self and to society, does not occur in its final form until all training is completed. Only then does the situation change from one of constant review by supervisors to one of peer and client review (Friedson, 1970). Specialists are certified twice, and this increases the importance of licensure as a social control mechanism (Bucher, 1970). The student becomes the healer and is viewed by others as the embodiment of the Hippocratic oath. This is a valued role in our society, which allows physicians to devalue their other roles. In Stryker's (1968) terms, the professional role has become paramount. With this internalization the professional socialization process is complete.

From this, it is evident that medical education provides the structures and cultural climate necessary to provide for a well-socialized independent practitioner at the end of the educational experience. The structures and the climate manage to overcome the emotional problems inherent in dealing with a field where error may mean death. The length of time of the socialization process and the candid recognition of the problems in the field allow the student to progress in an orderly, well-resolved sequence through the cognitive stages and to attain the final Stage IV of interdependence.

Appendix B

SUMMARY, HEW GRANT

A MULTI-VARIED ATTACK ON
ATTRITION AND STAFF-STUDENT RELATIONS

This 4-year project, designed to provide a multi-faceted attack on the problem of nursing student attrition, had two major goals:

1. Research into factors concomitant with success or attrition to discern causal patterns of behavior related to these variables.
2. Development and evaluation of an intervention program to reduce this attrition by providing both psychological and academic support services. Evaluation criteria used were graduation and attitudinal test results.

The program was instituted in a school of nursing that had experienced a student dropout rate ranging from 40%–60%, substantially higher than the national average. Intellectual inadequacy of the students could not have accounted for the high attrition. Based on entering NLN and ACT scores, all admitted students should have been able to complete the course. Analysis of exit interviews during the 5 years prior to 1968 had indicated that two factors, emotional problems and an inability to accept the demands of the nursing role, played a significant part in student withdrawal.

A pilot program offered two types of support services:

1. Crisis intervention: individual counseling for specific emotional problems in eight 1-hour sessions
2. Motivational groups: students in academic jeopardy could gain an understanding of the emotional basis for their underachievement.

A third service, remedial tutoring in math and reading, was added 6 months later when it became apparent that many emotionally stable, potentially capable students had been inadequately prepared for higher education.

The results of this pilot program were favorable. Students participating in either or both of the two psychological meliorative programs had a 21% attrition rate, compared to the 40% rate in a nontreatment control group.

An expanded 4-year project, which was to include a related program for the faculty and research into personality factors concomitant with student success or failure, was proposed to the HEW Nursing Demonstration and funded April 1, 1971.

It was theorized that the faculty program, consisting of consultation, teaching seminars, and T-groups, would strengthen the faculty's teaching skills and help promote emotional rapport with students, thereby reducing the number of students in need of treatment. Further, by expanding the program to include research into factors beyond the usual academic predictors, students in need of psychological support could be identified before the onset of either an emotional crisis or failing grades.

Although the action goals of the project were accomplished, the HEW project did not replicate the pilot studies' dramatic decrease in attrition. Attrition remained in the same 40%–60% range as a result of a completely altered administration, enrollment, and overall academic situation in the school.

Just prior to the entrance of the target class, a new administrative body took over the direction of the school, changing the organizational structure and, at least implicitly, the philosophy of education at the school. There was a drastic change in the composition of the class. Instead of 60 students, there were now 98. Now 42% of the class had NLN or ACT scores predicting certain failure. The change in the political atmosphere of the institution had further implications for the project besides the alteration of the class size and the sudden dramatic lowering of the predictor scores. The faculty became first apprehensive and then outraged at seeing their entrance standards overridden. Most of the students who would need the project's services were black or Latino, which created an appearance of racism and increased racial tensions.

The project exploring factors in attrition was also affected. Because of the faculty-student tensions, the target class was certain to have attitudinal profiles different from those of previous classes. To accomplish the research objectives, the various predictive tests were administered to classes in six other Chicago-area diploma schools of nursing. Despite these changes, the project achieved most of its objectives. Research into factors correlating with success showed the expected correlations between socioeconomic status and success. Typically, socioeconomic status does correlate well with success, but in this study the correlation was unusually high because, unlike most studies of professionals in training, our sample covered the entire socioeconomic range.

Besides these expected findings, two other tests emerged as valuable in predicting success: The Identity Scale (Sims) and the Image of Nursing (Haas). If a student's Identity Scale score indicated an individual who perceived herself as someone who can cope with life, express her emotions, and function in groups; and/or the Image of Nursing score revealed a conception of nursing as a profession that provides meaningful work, and revealed a negative view of the training as restrictive on autonomy and social life, the student was likely to succeed.

Crisis intervention was shown to be an effective and economical utilization of psychological services in nursing education.

Motivational groups, originally developed for underachievers (to eliminate their negative concept of self-as-learner) and previously demonstrated as being effective and economical with an underachieving population, proved to be effective and economical, although to a lesser degree, with culturally deprived students. The sample was small but the results were impressive. Inadequately prepared inner-city students can, with group techniques and remediation in basic skills, be motivated and prepared to survive a nurses' educational program at an attrition rate approximating that of the normative student.

The faculty support program, intended to strengthen teaching skills and build faculty-student rapport, could not be demonstrated to be successful. However, the program was effective in maintaining the faculty's performance in an atmosphere of confusion and tension.

Appendix C

SUMMARY OF TESTS USED

THE SIXTEEN PERSONALITY FACTOR TEST

The Sixteen Personality Test (16 P.F.) is a factor analytically developed personality questionnaire, designed to be a comprehensive measurement of the major dimensions of human personality in adults from 16 years to late maturity. Test authors are Drs. R.B. Cattell and H.W. Eber. The sixteen primary dimensions of the 16 P.F. are briefly indicated below:

Factor
A	Reserved, detached, critical, cool	Outgoing, warmhearted, easygoing
B	Less intelligent, concrete-thinking	More intelligent, abstract-thinking
C	Affected by feelings, emotionally less stable, easily upset	Emotionally stable, faces reality, calm
D	Humble, mild, obedient, conforming	Assertive, independent, aggressive, stubborn
E	Sober, prudent, serious, taciturn	Happy-go-lucky, heedless, gay, enthusiastic
F	Expedient, alone to self	Conscientious, persevering, staid, rule-bound
G	Shy, restrained, diffident, timid	Venturesome, socially bold, uninhibited, spontaneous
H	Tough-minded, self-reliant	Tender-minded, dependent, over-protected, sensitive
I	Trusting, adaptable, free of jealousy, easy to get along with	Suspicious, opinionated, hard to fool
J	Practical, careful, conventional, regulated by external realities, proper	Imaginative, wrapped up in inner urgencies, careless of practical matters, bohemian
K	Forthright, natural, artless, sentimental	Shrewd, calculating, worldly, penetrating

L   Placid, self-assured, confident,   Apprehensive, worrying,
    serene   depressive, troubled
M   Conservative, respecting estab-   Experimenting, critical, liberal,
    lished ideas, tolerant of traditional   analytical, free-thinking
    difficulties
N   Group-dependent, a "joiner,"   Self-sufficient, prefers making
    good follower   own decisions, resourceful
O   Casual, careless of protocol,   Controlled, socially precise, self-
    untidy, follows own urges   disciplined, compulsive
P   Relaxed, tranquil, torpid,   Tense, driven, overwrought, fretful
    unfrustrated

Four composite second-order scores are combined from the primary factors. They are rougher and some information is lost, but they do provide a convenient capsulized description of personality, frequently in meaningful categories closer to everyday parlance. The four principle second-order 16 P.F. composites are:

Anxiety: The score shows the level of anxiety in the commonly accepted sense, which may either be manifested for normal situational reasons or may be neurotic in origin, the score correlating with psychiatric evaluations of anxiety level.

Extraversion vs. Introversion: A high score indicates a socially outgoing, uninhibited person, good at making contacts; a low score indicates an introvert, both shy and self-sufficient.

Touch poise vs. responsive emotionality: A high score indicates an enterprising, decisive, imperturbable personality. A low score points to a person deeply sensitive, guided by emotions, and subject to more frustration and depression.

Independence vs. dependence: High scores indicate an aggressive, independent, self-directing person; low scores indicate a group-dependent, agreeable, passive personality.

IDENTITY SCALE

The Identity Scale (Henry and Sims, 1970) consists of 56 items that tap six dimensions involved in an individual's decisions about his or her identity. Each item is scored on a 1-7 scale (the middle point 4 is excluded). The higher the score (that is, the closer to 7), the higher the positive pole on any factor. The lower the score, the greater the negative pole on any factor. A factor score for an individual consists of the addition of all scores on all items in the factor divided by the number of items in the factor. (A few items are stated negatively and poles must be reversed when scoring.) The dimensions are:

1. Identity
   a. career
   b. group membership
   c. evaluation of self
   d. positive affectual experience
2. Expressivity and comfort in a social context
3. Individualistic expressivity
4. Integrity
5. Autonomy within social limits
6. Trust

The test was given under two different sets of instructions. The first had students describe their self-identity, that is, "myself as I really am." The second had students describe the "ideal nurse."

THE SENTENCE COMPLETION TEST

The Sentence Completion test, developed in conjunction with the Getzels-Jackson Gifted Adolescent project (1964), consists of 34 incomplete sentences that tap attitudes in four areas of concern to adolescents: work, family, peers, and self-image. The test can be coded for positive or negative attitudes in the four areas, or for categorical response (that is, common responses to a particular incomplete sentence stem or set of stems to explore problems in any of the areas).

THE THEMATIC APPERCEPTION TEST (TAT)

The TAT, developed by Morgan and Murray (1935), was adapted to explore the nursing student population's perception of issues that might be related to their choice of nursing as a profession and their potential nursing performance. Four standard cards (1, 3BM, 6BM, and 7GF) were used to tap issues and conflicts associated with achievement, depression, isolation, mother-child conflict, sibling rivalry, and independence. Four cards specially designed for this project were used to tap conflicts associated with the self-concept, reactions to female authority, and heterosexual intimacy. The cards can be scored so that individuals can be grouped according to their perceptions of the world and their views of conflict. These groupings were related to variables such as success in school, reaction to crises, maturity, and perceptions of the nursing field.

THE LIFE SPACE QUESTIONNAIRE

The Life Space questionnaire, patterned after a questionnaire on career women developed at National Opinion Research Center (1968), measures the female student nurse's perception of herself as a female in professional training.

THE IMAGE OF
NURSING SCALE QUESTIONNAIRE

The Image of Nursing Scale Questionnaire produced three typologies of attitudes toward the nursing profession, which are outlined in Chapter 6.

•••

In addition to these tests, the case studies in Chapter 9 included demographic data, intellectual ability, age, sex, race, and socioeconomic background. Intellectual ability was rated on variables that included decile of rank in high school class, the California Achievement Test in reading and math, the Iowa Test of Educational Development, the National League of Nursing Test (NLN), and the American College Testing (ACT) program.

Appendix D

ANNOTATED BIBLIOGRAPHY

GENERAL REFERENCES

Bradford, L.P., Gibb, J.R., and Benne, K.D. 1964. *T-Group Theory and Laboratory Method.* New York: John Wiley & Sons.

A detailed analysis of the general development and techniques of T-Group participation in which participants construct a group that will meet the requirements of all of its members for growth. T-Group training has five general aims: (a) a spirit of inquiry and willingness to experiment with alternatives; (b) an expanded awareness about people and interpersonal relations; (c) increased ability to reveal one's inner feelings without feeling compelled to play a role; (d) increased ability to act in collaborative ways with peers, superiors, and subordinates rather than in authoritarian or hierarchical terms; and (e) the ability to resolve conflict situations through problem solving rather than through coercion or manipulation.

Bucher, R., and Stelling, G. 1977. Becoming professional. *Sage Library of Social Research,* vol. 46. Beverly Hills: Sage Publications.

A comparative and longitudinal study that follows two cohorts of residents in psychiatry, one cohort of advanced students in biochemistry and one in internal medicine to provide data for a theory of professional socialization. Little support was found for the medical profession's claims that their socialization process builds effective mechanisms for individual self-control or colleague control among professionals. There is no way to determine whether professional claims of expertise correspond to real expertise. Suggestions to planners of professional training programs are offered.

Caplan, G. 1964. *Principles of Preventive Psychiatry.* New York: Basic Books, Inc.

A detailed analysis of the theory and practice of the preventive approach in the mental health field. A chief tool of prevention is consultation aimed at the professional having work-related difficulties. Four types of consultation are differentiated: (a) client-centered case consultation; (b) program-centered administrative consultation; (c) consultee-centered consultation; and (d) consultee-centered administrative consultation. Caplan describes the different techniques used for each type of consultation and how to choose the most appropriate type of consultation technique for a particular situation.

THE FIELD OF NURSING

American Nurses' Association. 1965. Position Paper on Nursing Education. In Bullough, B., and Bullough, V. (editors): *Expanding Horizons for Nurses.* 1977. New York: Springer Publishing Co., Inc.

The Nightingale ideal is upheld and nurses are urged to follow Nightingale's prescriptions. The present integration of nursing education into the hospital system is critically analyzed.

Batey, M.V. 1969. The Two normative worlds of the university nursing faculty. *Nursing Forum* 8(1):4-16.

University and hospital norms, goals, and reward systems are contrasted. Nurse faculty members are initially socialized into the norms, goals and rewards of the hospital, and no formal socialization is offered to counteract this initial training. Change in this situation might aid the expression of creativity, initiative, and self-direction by young faculty members, a change which would help the profession as a whole.

Benne, K.D., and Bennis, W. 1959. Role confusion and conflict in nursing: The role of the professional nurse. *American Journal of Nursing* 59:196-198.

Definitions of the social role of the professional nurse and points of conflict in these definitions are presented. Nurses in an outpatient department in a hospital were studied, and four principal sets of expectations that determine the character of the nurse's role were found: Official expectations stemming from the institution in which the nurse works; expectations of the nurse's immediate colleagues, subordinates, and peers in the working situation; expectations of the reference group outside the nurse's immediate work situation; and the nurse's own expectations of what a nurse should be and do.

Benne, K.D., and Bennis, W. 1959. Role confusion and conflict in nursing: What is real nursing? *American Journal of Nursing* 59:380-383.

Three of the principal areas of tension are examined: Frustration arising from the discrepancy between a nurse's image of "real" nursing and the functions she must assume in real work situations; the doctor-nurse relationship; and promotion, which often means conflict between a desire for higher status and a psychological need to give bedside care.

Nurses tend to reduce these conflicts by losing interest in their work, rationalizing away the conflicts, or organizing usually informal types of resistance to organizational demands. None of these strategies is seen as being conducive to the growth of the profession or of the professional.

Bullough, B. 1975. Factors contributing to role expansion for registered nurses. In Bullough, B. (editor): *The Law and the Expanding Nurse Role.* New York: Appleton Century Crofts, 53-61.

Several factors have contributed to the role expansion nurses have experienced in recent years: Educational changes have caused the decrease in diploma programs and the increase in collegiate programs, as well as the increasing importance of graduate education. A shortage of primary care physicians, caused by the trend toward greater specialization and the increased level of technology of medical equipment, has caused the amount of responsibility nurses must take for patient care to be expanded. The increasing use of physician's assistants paradoxically has helped the nurse practitioner movement by demonstrating to the public that some medical tasks can be delegated successfully. Two relevant societal trends are the women's liberation movement and the increasing number of elderly people with chronic illnesses. This last factor has helped expand the nurse's role because it is a problem for which nurses' training is more appropriate than physicians'.

Bullough, B., and Bullough, V., editors. 1977. *Expanding Horizons for Nurses.* Vol. III. New York: Springer Publishing Co., Inc.

Contains papers published between 1967 and 1976 dealing with the expanding professional functions of nurses, clinical controversies, legislative issues, nursing education, and women's liberation and nursing.

Brandt, E.M., Hastie, B., and Schumann, D. 1967. Comparison of on-the-job performance of graduates with school of nursing objectives. *Nursing Research* 16:50-60.

This study was designed to identify areas in which graduate nurses felt well-prepared and to provide data about aspects of their jobs that graduates considered to be in need of reinforcement. On the whole, the study group of B.S.N. nurses considered themselves to be as capable as or more capable than most graduate nurses and were also viewed as such by their immediate supervisors. The largest differences existed in the area of decision-making. This finding coincides with other reports in the literature.

Cleland, V. 1971. Sex discrimination: Nursing's most pervasive problem. *American Journal of Nursing* 71:1542-1547.

Sex discrimination is a frequent occurrence for nurses. For example, administrative positions in nursing are generally available only with the approval of the males in medicine, hospital administration, or higher education. The majority of directors of nursing do not control their own budgets, and faculty members in nursing are often paid less than male faculty members in other departments who have the same rank. Family roles and the nurse's role need to change. The admission of more men into nursing might alleviate some of these problems.

Corwin, R.C., Taves, M.J., and Haas, J.E. 1961. Professional disillusionment. *Nursing Research* 10:141-144.

The impression students have of nursing is not entirely realistic and leads to disillusionment after graduation. There is a fundamental disagreement about the role identity of the nurse as conceptualized by the schools of nursing, which endorse a professional orientation, and the medical-administrative hospital personnel, who expect the nurse to behave less professionally and more bureaucratically. Students are not fully prepared for the status transition to nurse in a hospital bureaucracy.

Grandjean, B.D., Aiken, L.H., and Bonjean, C.M. 1976. Professional autonomy and the work satisfaction of nursing educators. *Nursing Research* 25:216-221.

The importance and satisfaction associated with 21 characteristics of a nurse faculty position were examined. Teaching, supportive colleagues, keeping clinical knowledge current, and faculty autonomy were shown to be valued by faculty members. Increased professional autonomy would benefit faculty morale, recruitment, retention, and overall effectiveness in nursing education.

Group, T.M., and Roberts, J.I. 1974. Exorcising the ghosts of the Crimea. *Nursing Outlook* 22(6):368-372.

Faculty isolation, power plays, student isolation, and agency authority in nursing education are examined. The Crimean mentality that still prevails in nursing is authoritarian, militaristic, and male-dominated. The right of faculty women to be treated the same way as faculty men is asserted. Only when faculty members become part of the university mainstream will students be able to join with them. The questioning and bright students must not be labeled deviants or troublemakers, but efforts to engage them in intellectual inquiry should be initiated and sustained by both faculty and administration. Students, faculty, and administrators must all be involved in decision-making processes if this mentality is to be exorcised.

Harvey, L.H. 1970. Educational problems of minority group nurses. *Nursing Outlook* 18(9):48-50.

The dearth of nurses from the minority groups is reported. The main problems experienced by minority students are lack of relevant background in vital academic areas, cultural and income differences, anxiety from perceived isolation and exclusion, and unwillingness to meet standards imposed from a different cultural background. A successful program designed for large groups of minority students should include full information about the characteristics and demands of the specific educational program, a higher-than-average amount of financial assistance, and counseling on a comprehensive basis with generous empathetic support. They should be helped in every way possible to

internalize concepts of higher standards and see concrete examples of successful role models.

Johnson, M.M., and Martin, H.W. 1958. A Sociological analysis of the nurse role.
American Journal of Sociology 58(March):373-377.

Nursing is seen as an expressive rather than an instrumental role. This
means that nursing is related to "maintaining motivational equlibrium,"
rather than to moving something toward a goal. The claim is that physicians
are primarily instrumental while nurses are primarily expressive in the thera-
peutic environment. Thus the nurse must expedite the establishment and main-
tenance of harmonious relationships between physicians and patients. However, this expressiveness should not be taken too far, so that nurses get involved
emotionally with their patients.

Katz, F.E. 1969. Nurses. In Etzioni, A. (editor): *The Semi-Professions and Their
Organization*. New York: The Free Press, 54-81.

Professions are traditional guardians of bodies of knowledge, but nurses
are denied access to knowledge, which is controlled primarily by physicians.
The nurse acts as a buffer between the patient and the physician to protect the
physician and the hospital. Nurses also do not determine the kind of knowledge that is used in medical settings; their expertise is in behavioral science
knowledge, which is not even institutionalized into nursing theory. Hospitals
gain the loyalty of the thus de facto disenfranchised nurses by permitting them
to enact the nurturant care functions for patients.

Kramer, M. 1969. The new graduate speaks again. *American Journal of Nursing* 69(9):
1903-1907.

This study followed up an earlier study made on the initial work experience and feelings about nursing of 79 nurse subjects tested shortly after graduation. This study, conducted two years after graduation, found that continually employed nurses who had initially held high professional role conceptions
showed a significant decline in these values.

Rogers, M. 1972. Nursing: To be or not to be. *Nursing Outlook* 20(12)42-46.

Nursing has an identity and is a learned profession. "The science of nursing is not a summation of facts and principles drawn from other sources; it is a
science of synergistic man — unitary man — characterized by an organized conceptual system from which are derived the hypothetical generalizations and
unifying principles essential to guide practice." Nursing exists to serve society,
not the medical profession. The new programs for "physician's assistants"
and "pediatric associates" are scarcely disguised attempts by the medical
establishment to "gull registered nurses into leaving nursing to play handmaiden to medical mythology and machines." The distinction between professional and technical nurses is noted. "Only professionally educated nurses are
competent to guide nursing practice and to make the complex judgments that
require substantive knowledge and a high degree of intellectual skill . . . Bac-

calaureate graduates in nursing are not more interchangeable with associate degree and hospital graduates than dentists with dental hygienists or medical doctors with physician's assistants."

Schmitt, M.H. 1968. Role conflict in nursing. *American Journal of Nursing* 68:2348-2350.

This article examines nursing's current identity conflict, which stems from its attempt to maintain the "mothering" role while becoming professional. Nursing cannot turn back to the traditional images of the ministering angel if this means becoming any less professional and technically competent. Nursing must aim toward the "human side" of patient care. The ideal image of the nurse for the future is a special blending of the old and warm Nightingale spirit with the new and cold professional skills.

Stein, L.I. 1968. The doctor-nurse game. *American Journal of Nursing* 68:101-105.

The relationship between the physician and the nurse is seen as a game in which the nurse must subtly manipulate the doctor. Open disagreement is not permitted. The major disadvantage of a doctor-nurse game is its inhibitory effect upon dialogue. The game is basically a transactional neurosis, and both professions would be enhanced by a change in the attitudes that breed the game.

Williamson, J.A. 1972. The conflict-producing role of the professionally socialized nurse-faculty member. *Nursing Forum* II(4):356-366.

The organization of hospitals differs quite substantially from the organization of universities, and the organization of departments of nursing within universities is organized along lines that resemble the hospital structure. Thus, most decisions are made by the head of the department, even though this is not the norm in other university departments, which are much more collegial. This lack of autonomy experienced by nurse faculty members results from their original training in hospital situations, and has negative consequences for the profession and nursing students.

Wilson, V. 1971. An analysis of femininity in nursing. *American Behavioral Scientist* 15(2):213-220.

Although nursing is predominantly a female field, traditionally feminine elements of the nursing role must change if nursing is to become a professional field. Nurses are traditionally noted for their intuition rather than their intellect, for nurturance rather than productivity, and for dependency rather than independence. The second of these pairs will have to come to predominate.

CHARACTERISTICS OF NURSING STUDENTS

Adams, J. 1970. Considerations in assessing changes in personality characteristics of nursing students. *Journal of Psychiatric Nursing.* 8(4):12-16.

This study was designed to assess personality and attitudinal changes that might occur between the beginning and end of a psychiatric affiliation. Students in general medical hospital training and students in psychiatric affiliation were tested. The students in psychiatry modified their attitudes toward psychiatric patients, and students on the other rotations did not. The only significant difference between the two groups was in their change or lack of change toward psychiatric patients, although they experienced comparable change on several somewhat inconsistent variables. The significant change in both groups may indicate the reliability of the scales used.

Adams, J., and Klein, J.R. 1970. Students in nursing school: Considerations in assessing personality characteristics. *Nursing Research* 19:362-366.

This study compares the personalities of a current sample of nursing students with those of a comparable sample tested in 1959. The results indicate a number of changes that seem to parallel more general changes in attitudes seen in the nursing students' contemporaries.

Alutto, J.A., and others. 1971. A study of differential socialization for members of one professional occupation. *Journal of Health and Social Behavior* 12(June):140-147.

This study compared students from the three types of programs. Characteristics of senior nursing students selected for comparison purpose were professional commitment, organization commitment, clinical specialty commitment, role conflict, interpersonal trust, and authoritarianism. It was found that (a) the personality characteristics of students do differ, thereby ensuring variation in the general nursing population; and (b) regardless of any initial personality similarities or differences, graduating nurses from associate, diploma, and baccalaureate programs do not differ in terms of cognitive commitments to speciality areas.

Bailey, J.T. and Claus, K.E. 1969. Comparative analysis of the personality structure of nursing students. *Nursing Research* 18:320-326.

This report describes the personality patterns of four classes of nursing students in their sophomore year; compares the personality patterns of these nursing students with the "general college woman;" and compares the University of California nursing student with other nursing student groups. Analysis of variance on the mean raw scores on the EPPS revealed no marked differences among the entering classes of students. U.C. nursing students are markedly different from the general sample of college women. Nursing students from different institutions and different nursing education programs do not have identical need patterns as measured by the EPPS. All five groups of nursing students share only the need patterns of nurturance, order, abasement, and succorance.

Bayer, A.E. and Schoenfeldt, L.F. 1970. Student interchangeability in three-year and four-year nursing programs. *The Journal of Human Resources* 5(1):71-88.

This study analyzes measures of interests and personality, scores on aptitude and achievement tests, and data on personal and background variables using data from a national longitudinal survey that included first-year nursing students and recent nursing graduates. Generally negligible differences were found between students in three-year programs and those in four-year programs. No significant differences were found between the two groups in personality measures designed to assess temperament. With few exceptions, the interests of the two groups tended to be similar. Differences observed between groups tended to be in the domain of the arts and probably have little effect on one's role performance as a nurse. Family of orientation variables—status of siblings, family size—were not crucial in differentiating the groups. Socioeconomic background variables were among the primary differentiating variables of all those employed in the analysis. The second major set of variables that differentiated the two groups related to the college plans of the students and their parents' encouragement when they were enrolled in high school. These conclusions suggest that students currently completing three-year programs can perform as well as those who now enter and complete baccalaureate programs.

Christman, N.J. 1971. Clinical performance of baccalaureate graduates. *Nursing Outlook* 19(1):54-56.

The study was aimed at identifying the level of performance of baccalaureate graduate nurses employed in functional and unit-management patient care assignment settings. The seven components of nursing care, as defined by Krueter, were used in this study. Analysis of the subscores related to Kreuter's seven components led to identification of areas of nursing care provided at lower levels of performance by the baccalaureate graduates. The conclusions of the study lead to two primary recommendations for increasing the baccalaureate graduate's level of performance and the quality of care provided to hospitalized patients: the method of providing nursing care must center on the patient as an individual, and nursing care seminars for staff nurses and head nurses should be instituted to improve the nurse's performance within this method of providing patient care.

Cleveland, S.E. 1961. Personality patterns associated with the professions of dietitian and nurse. *Journal of Health and Human Behavior* 2:113-124.

The personality characteristics, as revealed by the Thematic Apperception Test, of dietitian and nurse groups at both the student and staff levels are compared. Compared to dietetic interns, nursing students scored significantly higher on passivity themes, use of distress words and sad-lonely words, and negative parental attitudes, and scored lower on achievement and positive parental attitudes. Staff members' scores showed similar trends but to a lesser degree.

Corwin, R.G. 1961. The professional employee: A study of conflict in nursing roles. *Sociological Perspectives on Occupations,* ed. R.M. Pavalko, p. 261-275.

This study investigated whether bureaucratic and professional conceptions of the role of nurse produce conflict, whether there are systematic differences in the organization of roles produced by diploma and degree programs, and whether the discrepancies between ideal role and perceptions of the reality increase after graduation. Bureaucratic and professional conceptions of role, jointly held, prevent adequate fulfillment of either role. Degree nurses maintain high professional conceptions more frequently than do diploma nurses, combining them with either high or low bureaucratic conceptions. This simultaneous allegiance to both roles suggests the intensity of the conflict they encounter. Although degree nurses are unlikely to hold high bureaucratic and low professional conceptions, this is a popular choice among diploma nurses. However, the conceptual organization of diploma and degree *students* does not differ. After graduation, degree nurses also frequently attempt to combine professional conception with high bureaucratic conception, which probably increases the conflict. Diploma nurses express lower professional and service conceptions of role than diploma students do, suggesting that these are modified after graduation while bureaucratic conceptions are apparently maintained. On the other hand, among degree nurses the professional conception seems to be maintained after graduation, while the bureaucratic conception increases after graduation.

Davis, A.J. 1969. Self-concept, occupational role expectations, and occupational choice in nursing and social work. *Nursing Research* 18:55-59.

This study explored the differences in the self-concept and occupational role expectations of women students in nursing and social work. Most social work students described themselves as independent, spontaneous, and assertive. The nursing students' self-concept was best described as dependable, methodical, capable, and conscientious, with some tendency to be submissive and to sustain subordinate roles.

Dustan, L.C. 1964. Characteristics of students in three types of nursing education programs. *Nursing Research* 13:159-166.

The purpose of this study was to determine the "fit" between the requirements and objectives of each of the three types of programs and the characteristics and career expectations of the enrolled students. On the basis of scholastic aptitude, values, interests, and long-range career plans, the associate-degree students were judged inappropriately matched with the objectives and curriculum requirements of a program designed to be a terminal offering at the lower division level. The students in the diploma programs were judged to be well matched to their less scientifically oriented curricula, which placed major emphasis on direct care to patients in a hospital setting. Differences among the groups were found only in age and marital status; differences in ability and interest patterns were marginally significant.

Edwards, C.N. 1963. Cultural dissonance and dissimulation: A study in role conflict. *Journal of Consulting and Clinical Psychology* 32:607-610.

The study tested the hypotheses that the perception of cultural dissonance in the career-marriage matrix is positively related to dissimulation and that this negative relationship will be greater among women showing a preference for compromise roles. A "career-oriented" population differed significantly from the "compromise group" in the predicted direction. However, significant difference between the two populations makes it impossible to draw any firm conclusions about the relationships within the combined group because teachers' well-being is negatively related to career commitment, and nurses' well-being is positively related to career commitment.

Gortner, S.R. 1968. Nursing majors in twelve western universities: A comparison of registered nurse students and basic senior students. *Nursing Research* 17:121-128.

This study attempts to describe values, personality characteristics, educational and professional motivations, and socioeconomic origins of R.N. students. It also attempts to differentiate the R.N. student from the senior nursing student in the basic collegiate program. The data supported the theory that R.N. students have a greater professional orientation. However, the groups did not differ in personality, interest patterns, or career choice patterns. The R.N. students come from families with lower social standing than the B.S.N. students, and upward mobility was a factor in their career choice.

Hover, J. 1975. Diploma vs. degree nurses: Are they alike? *Nursing Outlook* 23(11):684-687.

The purpose of this study was to determine whether goals and attitudes about nursing differed as a result of the type of basic nursing education the nurse had experienced. Nurses were found to differ according to their educational preparation. Compared to diploma graduates, degree graduates are less restricted in patient preferences, place higher value on ability and lower value on personal traits as characteristics typifying good nurses, show more satisfaction with their education, and seem more likely to seek promotions outside the hospital system. Diploma graduates working toward degrees in nursing hold opinions and goals approaching those of degree graduates.

Ingmire, A.E. 1952. Attitudes of student nurses at the University of California. *Nursing Research* 1:36-39.

This study investigated attitudes that may influence the progress of students in nursing. The areas of home and family relationships, personal relationships, nursing activities, and future plans and aspirations were selected as being particularly important in the nursing students' progress. Attitudes toward family members were, on the whole, good. Students felt secure in the love and affection of their parents. Students were free from problems concerning finance, health, social and personal relationships, and religion. The majority said they were happy in nursing, were receiving a good professional education, and were able to give good care to patients. They participated in extracurricular activities. They recognized their community and social responsibilities. All students expressed negative attitudes in one or more areas of their nursing experience. First-year students enjoyed the majority of their classes and liked their head nurses but expressed ambivalent attitudes toward supervision.

Second-year students were highly sensitive, had easily hurt feelings, and feelings of inferiority to other students, graduate nurses, and the medical staff. Their dissatisfactions were more generalized. They were more critical of evaluations of their work, of instruction, and of personnel. Third-year students had even less security in their status as active team members, said their work was directed by physicians and reported that they had little responsibility for assisting in planning care. The ideals of service held on admission gave way to a conviction that nursing is a job—a "never ending job."

Johnson, R.W., and Leonard, L.C. 1970. Psychological test characteristics and performance of nursing students. *Nursing Research* 19:147-150.

The purposes of this study were to describe the psychological characteristics of students beginning the professional course sequence in a baccalaureate nursing program and to determine the effectiveness of these characteristics in predicting theory and practice grades. Students with a good background in math, high abstract reasoning ability, high academic motivation, and low sales interests were most likely to obtain high theory grades. In contrast, the test scores were of very little value in predicting grades. The final grades (theory and practice grades combined) were best predicted by abstract reasoning ability.

Levitt, E.E., Lubin, B., and Zuckerman, M. 1962. The student nurse, the college woman, and the graduate nurse: A comparative study. *Nursing Research* 11:80-82.

This study measured the consistency of the nursing student pattern over several years, compared the nursing student pattern with that of the general college woman, and compared nursing students with graduate nurses tested by Navran and Stauffacher (1957). The Edwards Personal Preference Schedule was used. In the characteristic personality pattern of needs prior to the clinical years in nursing school, masculine needs such as autonomy, dominance, and aggression, are deemphasized. The less assertive, more feminine needs, such as succorance, nurturance, and abasement, predominate. Nursing students may exhibit an accentuation of the feminine social need pattern with nurturance as the pinnacle.

McDonald, T.D. and others. 1969. Occupational choice, commitment, values, and orientations of nursing students. *Indian Sociological Bulletin* 7(1):1-11.

This project studied social and other variables affecting the decision to enter nursing: the sources of encouragement for nursing students, self-reported reason for choosing nursing, expectations of nursing, the relationship between the age of definite decision to enter nursing and doubts and seriousness of doubts about the decision to enter nursing, the age at which the respondents first thought of becoming a nurse and the doubts and the seriousness of doubts about the choice, years in nursing school, and commitment to discipline and career. Sources of influence on career choice were parental influence, employment opportunities, occupational contact, and peer group. There was a strong similarity between the sources of influence and the sources of encouragement. The majority of the respondents entered nursing to "help people and work with people."

Meleis, A.I., and Farrell, K.D. 1974. Operation concern: A study of senior nursing students in three nursing programs. *Nursing Research* 23:461-468.

The focus of this study was biographical and attitudinal differences and/or similarities among graduating seniors in the three different types of nursing education. Students in the three types of programs were found to be essentially alike on intellectual characteristics, the consideration aspect of leadership, and self-esteem. Compared to other college students, they were slightly above average in their concern for the feelings and welfare of people and were inclined to be affiliative, trusting, and ethical. They expressed similar degrees of consideration for subordinates and were inclined to respect their ideas. Baccalaureate students rated higher in the area of communication than associate degree or diploma seniors, and they were higher on the structure and autonomy factors of leadership. Diploma students placed highest value on research; baccalaureate students, lowest.

O'Mahoney, M.T., and Cohen, H.A. 1974. A typological analysis of personality and attitudinal profiles of student nurses. Unpublished paper. HEW Grant.

This study attempted to explain personality and attitudinal dimensions of nurses. The 16 P.F. Questionnaire and the Image of Nursing Scale were the scales used with these results: Contrary to earlier predictions, there is no single stereotypic nursing personality or single stereotypic view of the nursing field. Certain relationships between types of attitudes toward nursing and the different personality typologies were found. Most significantly, the expressive view of nursing was held by individuals who could be characterized as neurotic introverts. The instrumental view was held by individuals who fit into the modal personality typology.

Reichow, R.W., and Scott, R.E. 1976. Study compares graduates of two-, three-, and four-year programs. *Hospitals* 50:95-100.

The abilities of graduates of the three types of nursing education programs were compared. The data revealed that the larger institutions had a higher regard for the baccalaureate graduates than the smaller ones did, although both have a high opinion of diploma nurses. The hospitals rated the baccalaureate nurses higher in their knowledge of administrative procedures and equal to diploma nurses in leadership ability and in their ability to learn new concepts. Hospital administrators think a nurse is a nurse if she can get the job done.

Richards, M.A. 1972. A study of differences in psychological characteristics of students graduating from three types of basic nursing programs. *Nursing Research* 21:259-261.

The purpose of this study was to find any statistically significant differences in intelligence; levels of various personality characteristics such as leadership potential, responsibility, emotional stability, and sociability; or degree of professionism among graduates of associate degree, diploma, and baccalaureate degree nursing programs. No statistically significant differences were found among three groups of graduating students in leadership potential (ascendency), responsibility, emotional stability, or sociability. Diploma students showed the highest levels of leadership potential and sociability, and associate degree students demonstrated the highest levels of responsibility and emotional stability. Differences in intelligence were not significant at the .05 level; however, graduating diploma students had higher intelligence scores than the graduating associate degree students ($p > .10$). In describing their ideal of nursing practice, graduating baccalaureate students had a significantly ($p > .05$) more professional orientation than diploma and associate degree students.

Smith, J.E. 1968. Personality structure in beginning nursing students: A Factor analytic study. *Nursing Research* 17:140-145.

The personality inventory scores of a large group of nursing students were administered at each school. The scores of each student were analyzed by computer, resulting in the derivation of seven factors from the 21 variables of the tests. The factors were tenderhearted, strong-willed, religous-mystic, humble-religious, dependent-achiever, intellectual-achiever, and abasive-dependent. Some of these dimensions appear to incorporate characteristics that one would consider facilitating to the nursing role. Some may lead to success more than others. Educational implications inherent in the personality characteristics are suggested.

Stromberg, M. 1976. Relationship of sex role identity to occupational image of female nursing students. *Nursing Research* 25:363-369.

This study investigated the relationship between sex role identity, measured by the Masculinity-femininity (Mf) scale of Minnesota Multiphasic Personality Inventory (MMPI), and image of nursing, measured by Frank's 1969 Image of Nursing Questionnaire (INQ). A secondary purpose of the study was to determine if identifiable groups in the student population differed in their image of nursing. There is a relationship between nursing students' sex role identity and image of nursing. As the student's sex role identity became more masculine, the student's image of nursing was more in harmony with the image advanced by the profession. The image of nursing held by B.S.N. and A.D. students was higher (that is, more professional) than that of diploma students; there were no significant differences between the B.S.N. and A.D. students in this area.

SOCIALIZATION IN NURSING

Brown, J.S., Swift, Y.B., and Oberman, M.L. 1974. Baccalaureate students' images of nursing: A replication. *Nursing Research* 25:53-59.

A replication of the Davis and Olesen (1964) study. The findings lend support to the assumptions of Davis and Olesen that collegiate nursing stu-dents are recruited from a common pool of applicants, similar in social back-ground, aspirations, and beliefs. These students achieved less consensus than the students in Davis and Olesen's sample, but shared the humanistic and pro-fessional, rather than bureaucratic views expressed by the earlier sample.

Crocker, L.M., and Brodie, B.J. 1974. Development of a scale to assess student nurses' views of the professional nursing role. *Journal of Applied Psychology* 59(2):233-235.

The primary objective of this study was to construct a homogeneous scale to measure the congruence between nursing students' perceptions and faculty views of the professional nursing role. Results show a definite trend in student endorsement of the faculty view of the profession as graduation nears. This may indicate that the students' views are molded by actual clinical experi-ences, or that the faculty members who teach students basic skills and proce-dures also indoctrinate them with their own professional views.

Davis, F., and Olesen, V.L. 1964. Baccalaureate students' images of nursing. *Nursing Research* 13:8-15.

An examination of the images of nursing and their bearing on students' personal values. The findings are as follows: A pronounced trend towards individualistic and innovative images of nursing and away from bureaucratic images and a minor and inconsistent trend away from lay images of nursing; a commensurate increase in the personal importance students attach to individ-ualistic-innovative images, but at the same time no appreciable change in the importance they continue to attach to lay images; the teaching emphases of nursing faculty appear to exercise a considerable influence on the students' increasing endorsement of individualistic-innovative orientations, but such influence does not extend to all professional values that faculty claim to emphasize in their contacts with students; no significant overall increase in consensus among students in their characterizations of nursing or the per-sonal importance they attach to such characterizations; and no evidence that, on the average, students grow less "dissonant" in terms of reconciling their images of nursing with personal values.

Davis, F., and Olesen, V.L. 1965. The career outlook of professionally educated women. *Psychiatry* 28(4):334-345.

The focus of the study was to determine whether, and how, professional education in nursing influences the student's basic attitudes toward, and image of, work in relation to women's roles. Included were the relative value of work, the meanings attached toward work generally and nursing in particular, the quality of commitment to nursing, and general views on the situation of American women. A professional education in nursing in no way alters the fundamentally conventional orientation to the adult female role that these stu-dents brought with them initially. When asked to rank from four different attributes commonly associated with the adult female role, majorities of students rank "work and career" second, after first selecting "home and family." There was no increase in the proportion doing so from time of entry to graduation.

Davis, F., and Olesen, V.L. 1963. Initiation into a women's profession: Identity problems in the status transition of coed to student nurse. *Sociometry* 26(1):89-101.

What happens when aspirations to a profession lack one or more commitment-generating attributes? It was found that nursing students experience considerable identity stress because of the difficulty they have in psychologically integrating the nursing student role with a concurrently emerging identity of adult womanhood.

Edwards, C.N. 1969. The student nurse: A study in sex role transition. *Psychological Reports* 25:975-990.

The interaction of individual and institution within the nursing profession is explored. Of primary interest are the personality and motivational factors contributing to the selection of nursing as a profession, and the impact of the school of nursing and hospital setting on the progressive development of the student. Although drawing on empirical research, the paper is intended not as a presentation of empirical data but as a discussion of a social and psychological process. The academic and social structure is examined along with recruitment and motivation, socialization, personality, affiliations, and transition. One of the great challenges facing the professions in the future will be the development of a productive program to utilize the talents and contributions of nursing students, while at the same time providing a productive and socially acceptable way to negotiate adolescence.

Eisenman, R. 1970. Creativity change in student nurses: A cross-sectional and longitudinal study. *Developmental Psychology* 3(3):320-325.

This studies the change in creativity during nursing education. Two creativity measures were employed: Originality was measured by an unusual uses test, and creativity was measured by a true-false, paper-and-pencil measure, the Personal Opinion Survey. The originality scores derived from the unusual uses test indicated a decline in originality with increasing class standing. The longitudinal data are consistent with the cross-sectional results. The Personal Opinion Survey shows little change. Again, the longitudinal findings are fairly consistent with the cross-sectional data.

Eron, L.D. 1955. The Effect of nursing education on attitudes. *Nursing Research* 4:24-27.

This project studied changes in specific attitudes felt to be important in the nurse's work and in work gratification during the nursing school period. The authoritarianism, conservatism, cynicism, humanitarianism, and anxiety of each individual were studied, and a consistent trend for the more advanced students to receive lower scores on the authoritarianism scale was found.

There were no differences in scores on political-economic conservatism. Although third-year nurses received higher anxiety scores than first-year nurses, the difference in mean score was not statistically significant. On the cynicism and humanitarianism scales, the more advanced students secured significantly lower mean scores than did the beginning students.

Grissum, M., and Spengler, C. 1976. *Womanpower and Health Care.* Boston: Little, Brown and Co., Inc.

The process by which women health care professionals have traditionally been relegated to secondary status is explored and related to the societal forces that condition females to be passive, dependent, and indecisive. Women must learn to accept and use strategies associated with societal change to develop a sense of self-esteem and control over their lives.

Gunter, L.M. 1969. The developing nursing student (part II): Attitudes toward nursing as a career. *Nursing Research* 18:131-136.

Selected attitudes toward nursing as a career held by sophomore nursing students are described. Motivation toward nursing as a career was found to be very strong. Nursing students' ideal image of nursing is similar to that described in other reports. This motivation to help others, and to be virtually certain that actions will achieve the desired results and that no serious consequences will arise from mistakes, may preclude or impede the development of a professional person who holds a desire for independent action, is willing to experiment, to raise questions, and to assume responsibility without depending on a higher authority.

Jacox, A. 1973. Professional socialization of nurses. *Journal of the New York State Nurses Association* 4(4):6-15.

A discussion of the socialization of nursing without empirical data. The three core characteristics of professionalism—education, service, and autonomy—are discussed. Jacox concludes that it is necessary to encourage nurses to be more aggressive, individually and collectively, in taking those actions necesary for nurses to become more autonomous and self-directive.

Kohnke, M.F. 1973. Do nursing educators practice what is preached? *American Journal of Nursing* 73:1571-1578.

This study aimed at discovering whether educators were, in fact, producing two different products—nurse technician and professional nurse. The study compared what the literature stated was the knowledge base, responsibility, and role in the curricular preparation of the nurse technician and the professional nurse to the actual goals of deans of A.D. and B.S.N. programs. In practice, what the schools taught and faculty members perceived about the technical programs differed from what the literature stated. This also held true for the professional program. Few of the differences stated in the literature existed.

Mauksch, H.O. 1963. Becoming a nurse: A selective view. *Annals of the American Academy of Political and Social Sciences* 346:88-98.

The factors that affect the development of the young woman who enters a school of nursing and the impact on adolescents of the reality of contact with illness and death were examined. Students exhibited high needs for security, social control, and idealism; and held the traditional conception of nurse as one who helps people. The curricula and the educational philosophy of nursing are generally patient-centered and patient-directed. However, the traditional conception of nursing as the nurturant mother-surrogate has given way to several possible alternatives: the healing function, the coordinating function of unit management within the hospital structure, and the emergence of the patient-care oriented nurse clinician. The implication is that conflict could be expected to result from these changes.

May, W.T., and Ilardi, R.L. 1970. Image and stability of values of collegiate nursing students. *Nursing Research* 19:359-361.

The purpose of this study was to investigate value changes among nursing students during their educational experience. Findings suggest that there was a significant decrease in mean scores on the religious value scale and an increase in mean scores on the aesthetic value scale of the Allport-Vernon Lindzey Study of Values. Few other changes were found.

Moody, P.M. 1973. Attitudes of cynicism and humanitarianism in nursing students and staff nurses. *The Journal of Nursing Education* 12:9-13.

A comparison of attitudes of cynicism and humanitarianism in first-year nursing students, senior nursing students, and practicing nurses to discover whether nurses' attitudes of cynicism and humanitarianism change during their nursing school experience and after nursing school. The resulting data indicated no significant difference in humanitarianism scores between first-year nursing students and senior nurses, and that nurses' attitudes of cynicism are not changed during or after nursing school.

Olesen, V.L., and Davis, F. 1966. Baccalaureate students' images of nursing: A follow-up report. *Nursing Research* 15:151-158.

In this study, students came increasingly to characterize nursing and what they valued in it in terms of advanced professional images of the field. Complementary to this trend, a larger proportion of them came to reject bureaucratic images of the field, although a fair number continued to hold on to certain lay images. Despite these trends, students did not achieve greater consensus among themselves concerning what they believed does and does not characterize nursing. They did reach higher consensus on what in nursing they viewed as important or not important for the self. Except for their increasing endorsement of advanced professional images for both nursing and self, there was not a close correspondence between what they saw in nursing and the qualities of nursing they valued.

O'Neill, M.F. 1973. A study of baccalaureate nursing student values. *Nursing Research* 22:437-443.

The major purpose of this study was to compare the values of nursing students with other student groups at successive class levels in the nursing programs. The nursing students differed significantly from the general college female students on five of six of the interpersonal values. The nursing students placed greater emphasis on being generous and helping the unfortunate, and placed less emphasis on following rules closely. Students in the three schools differed from each other and thus changed in different ways.

Psathas, G. 1969. The fate of idealism in nursing school. *Journal of Health and Social Behavior* 9:52-64.

This paper explores the nursing students' perceptions and attitudes in relation to specific roles and situations. Freshmen express a degree of idealism and optimism not found among seniors. Freshmen also show greater concern with the problems and difficulties of nursing practice, relationships with patients, and problems faced in nursing school. Seniors give more "technique oriented" than "patient-centered" care, see patients more as "disease entities" than "whole" people with distinct personalities, and devote less energy toward meeting patient needs in a creative and distinctive fashion.

Redden, J.W., and Scales, E.E. Nursing education and personality characteristics. *Nursing Research* 10:215-218.

The purpose of the study was to determine if certain personality variables were subject to change during the freshman through senior years of nursing school and if the personality characteristics of black female nursing students differed from the normative college women described by Edwards. It was found that there were significant differences between mean scores of the normative group of college women and nursing students on 12 of the 15 variables. This group of nursing students had strong tendencies to defer, accept, analyze the whims and feelings of others, to judge others by why they act rather than by their actions, to help, assist, and support others, and to be aggressive. Few differences were found between classes in the sample.

Rubin, H.S., and Cohen, H.A. 1974. Group counseling and remediation: A two-faceted intervention approach to the problem of attrition in nursing education. *Journal of Educational Research* 67:195-198.

An investigation of the effectiveness of brief group therapy for under-achievement and of remediation for deficiencies in basic skills in reducing the attrition rate of 69 female student nurses. Students whose entering California Test of Achievement scores or GPAs indicated risk of academic failure were interviewed; those with high scores but with motivational problems (under-achievers) received appropriate therapy, those with low scores and no motivational problems received remediation, and those with low scores plus motivational problems received both. Results indicate a significant decrease in attrition rate.

Schoeberle, E.A., and Craddick, R.A. 1968. Human figure drawings by freshman and senior student nurses. *Perceptual and Motor Skills* 27:11-14.

The purpose of this study was to investigate the ideal-nurse image that nursing students at the freshman and senior levels have. The general results seem consistent with previous reports, which suggest that nursing students' attitudes, images, and concepts change from year to year as a function of their level of training. However, in view of the significant differences in ages between freshman and senior groups, one cannot rule out the possibility of simple maturity differences. One might speculate that seniors, who rated themselves closer to the "ideal" nurse than the freshman students, may consider themselves past most of the obstacles in training that could label them as undesirable and result in their being dropped from the program. This speculation gains some support in the findings that seniors drew the "undesirable" nurse larger than freshmen, perhaps indicating more distance from this image and permitting the seniors playfully to produce larger figures.

Schulz, E.D. 1965. Personality traits of nursing students and faculty concepts of desirable traits: A longitudinal comparative study. *Nursing Research* 14:261-264.

This paper studies personality changes in baccalaureate nursing students. For the class of 1961, significant differences were found for three variables on the EPPS, abasement, nurturance, and exhibition. For the class of 1962, there were ten significantly high mean difference scores: autonomy, heterosexuality, nurturance, deference, aggression, abasement, endurance, change, and succorance. For the class of 1963, there were eight significantly high mean difference scores: heterosexuality, autonomy, abasement, aggression, endurance, deference, nurturance, and achievement. There was very little relationship between faculty desirability ranking of the 15 traits from the EPPS and the performance of either group of students (sophomore or senior) on the EPPS.

Segal, B.E. 1962. Male nurses: A case study in status contradiction and prestige loss. *Social Forces* 41:31-38.

This study looks at the status contradiction and prestige loss of the male nurse. Male nurses are suspect because they enter a traditionally female occupation. They fail to meet the expectations that are supposed to govern men's career choices, because they exhibit a contradiction between characteristics ascribed to men in our society and characteristics ascribed to members of the nursing profession. The effect of this contradiction is that a man's prestige and self-esteem may suffer when he is in an occupation that is staffed mostly by women. By several measures, male and female nurses have approximately the same prestige rank; but male nurses feel as if they have the lower position, and the female nurses' statements corroborate the men's impressions.

Sharp, W.H., and Anderson, J.C. 1972. Changes in nursing students' descriptions of the personality traits of the ideal nurse. *Measurement and Evaluation in Guidance* 5:339-344.

This study tested the hypothesis that as nursing students progress through their educational programs, their descriptions of the personality traits of the ideal nurse will become progressively more similar to the faculty's descriptions of the ideal nurse. A secondary purpose of the study was to determine if successful and unsuccessful freshman nursing students differed in their descriptions of the ideal nurse. Cross-sectional data showed the largest differences between faculty and freshmen and fewer differences between the faculty and the other classes.

Siegel, H. 1968. Professional socialization in two baccalaureate programs. *Nursing Research* 17:403-407.

This study assessed the degree to which professional socialization occurred in two baccalaureate nursing education programs. Seniors' perceptions of nursing and related values were found to correspond closely with those of faculty members. Students assigned greater personal importance to advanced professional characteristics at later stages in both programs but did not typically attribute these characteristics to their picture of nursing. In general, student and faculty groups in the two programs did not differ in their attribution of advanced professional characteristics to nursing or in their valuation of these characteristics. Student groups reached greater consensus on the personal importance of the suggested characteristics of nursing, but not regarding what they saw in nursing. Individually, students did not typically achieve greater consonance within themselves between what they attributed to nursing and what they valued for themselves.

Tetreault, A.I. 1976. Selected factors associated with professional attitudes of baccalaureate nursing students. *Nursing Research* 25:49-53.

This paper examined the correlation between professional attitude and selected situational and demographic factors of baccalaureate nursing students. Professional attitudes were found to be highest for students 24 to 26 years of age, who saw nursing as highly positive and highly active, who had the largest number of formal and informal nursing experiences, and whose teachers were seen as trustworthy and professional. Professional attitude of students was not associated significantly with potency attributed to nursing, career choice, parents' level of education, or placement in sibling group.

Ventura, M.R., and Meyers, C.R. 1976. Creative thinking abilities of student nurses. *Psychological Reports* 39:409-410.

This study compared creative thinking abilities of senior nursing students in associate degree, diploma, and baccalaureate degree programs. Results of the Torrance Test of Creative Thinking, Form A, revealed that diploma nursing students scored significantly higher on Verbal Fluency than the other groups; diploma nursing students earned significantly higher scores on Figural Fluency and Figural Flexibility than baccalaureate degree students; baccalaureate degree students scored significantly higher on Verbal Originality than the others; and significant differences appeared between all groups on Figural Elaboration with associate degree students scoring the highest and diploma students the lowest. The only nonsignificant differences disclosed were for Verbal Flexibility and Figural Originality. These findings may be attributed to such factors as: emphasis on liberal arts in college nursing programs, sampling procedure, and differences existing between students in their respective programs prior to entrance to nursing school.

Werner, M.A. 1973. Professional socialization of nurses: A faculty member's view. *Journal of the New York State Nurses' Association* 4(4):21-23.

The influence teachers have on the students in terms of professional socialization is examined. Students observe the faculty very closely, not only in the classroom or clinical setting, but in the halls, coffee shop, cafeteria, meetings, and at student-faculty social affairs. Anything a student learns about the faculty — good or bad — stands a chance of becoming incorporated into that student's value system. This is the challenge for faculty in professional socialization.

Williams, T.R., and Williams, M.M. 1959. The socialization of the student nurse. *Nursing Research* 8:18-25.

The research reported here focuses on the kinds of techniques used to elicit behavior and attitude expressions from the nursing student that leads her to general conformity to the ideals held by her instructors. Three techniques — the Nightingale ideal, the rationale of science, and the authoritarian control — and their corollaries appear to be the basic means by which the nursing instructors in five diverse schools lead students to exhibit the behavior and attitudes considered necessary for a graduate professional nurse.

PREDICTORS OF SUCCESS IN NURSING

Hutcheson, J.D., Garland, L.M., and Prather, J.E. 1973. Toward reducing attrition in baccalaureate degree nursing programs: An exploratory study. *Nursing Research* 22:530-533.

An attempt to identify some of the causes of attrition in baccalaureate degree programs. The study included 73 demographic, academic, and program-related variables. A principal component factor analysis resulted in five factors — nursing school performance, scholastic aptitude, demographic characteristics, scholastic achievement, and socioeconomic status — which accounted for 50% of the total variance. These factors were used to provide a set of indicator variables that were subsequently correlated with attrition. Demographic characteristics and academic aptitude and achievement did not prove to be reliable in identifying potential dropouts. The only variable that correlated strongly with completion was a composite clinical evaluation.

Katzell, M.E. 1968. Expectations and dropouts in schools of nursing. *Journal of Applied Psychology* 52(2):154-157.

This study was undertaken as a partial test of the March and Simon theory, as applied to withdrawal from schools of nursing. The theory predicts that the greater the number of satisfactions experienced, the more likely a student will be to continue in a school of nursing. In Katzell's study, students who remained in school had experienced more satisfaction. The survivors had significantly more of their expectation confirmed than did the dropouts. The nonacademic and total dropout groups exceeded survivors in numbers of satisfactions that were neither expected nor experienced. No relationship was demonstrated in any of the groups between withdrawal and either expected satisfactions, expected stresses, experienced stresses, expected stresses that were experienced, unexpected stresses that were experienced, and unexpected stresses that were not experienced.

Kelly, W.L. 1974. Psychological prediction of leadership in nursing. *Nursing Research* 23:38-42.

This study investigated whether personality tests have enough discriminatory power to be able to predict those who were actually promoted and those who were evaluated for promotion but not promoted, either because they did not qualify or because there were not sufficient positions available for all who qualified for promotion. The decisive traits of the promoted nurses were found to be capacity for status, femininity, a relaxed demeanor, independence, distance, and a lower propensity for stress.

Kibrick, A.K., and Tiedeman, D.V. 1961. Conceptions of self and perception of role in schools of nursing. *Journal of Counseling Psychology* 8(1):62-69.

This study considered adjustments that must be made to vocational decisions once such decisions have been acted upon. The hypothesis tested was that the more the students' expectations matched those of their instructors upon entrance, the more likely those students would be to complete their education. However, the results suggest that, at entry, incompatibility with instructors' expectations does not have a marked influence upon a student leaving school within 6 months.

Krueger, C. 1968. Do bad girls become good nurses? *Trans-Action* 5(July):31-36.

An investigation of the relationship between virtue and being a good nurse. The rules, the right attitude, and the right moral reputation had something to do with being a good nursing student but very little to do with being a good working nurse.

Michael, W.B., and others. 1971. The criterion-related validities of cognitive and non-cognitive predictions in a training program for nursing candidates. *Educational and Psychological Measurement* 31(Winter)983-987.

The study demonstrated that a cognitive measure (the California Reading Test) and highschool grades were the most valid predictors for success of nursing school candidates. Personality factors, as derived from the 16 P.F. and the MMPI, did not prove to be adequate predictors of success, nor did a test of spatial visualization.

O'Mahoney, M., and Labbie, S. 1973. Factors of the image of nursing scale and their relation to personality dimensions and GPA. Presented at American Psychological Association Annual Meeting, Montreal.

This study attempts to isolate more specific dimensions of a student's attitude concerning nursing and to relate these dimensions to an index of academic success. Students who hold a positive image of the field, who view nurses as more intelligent, better educated, and more respected than women in other professions, tend to do well academically. These students view nursing as an appropriate field of endeavor for persons such as themselves, and this congruence seems to function as an additional motivating factor. Students who perceive nursing as offering greater personal and financial independence and an interesting future view themselves as self-sufficient, outgoing, and emotionally stable, and also tend to perform well academically. Factors of "worthwhile service," "cost of education," and "secondary benefits," such as the opportunity to put one's religious beliefs into practice, were not related to academic success.

Owen, S.V., Feldhusen, J.F., and Thurston, J.R. 1970. Achievement prediction in nursing education with cognitive, attitudinal, and divergent thinking variables. *Psychological Reports* 26:867-870.

This study attempted to determine whether two attitude measures, designed for prediction of achievement in nursing education, and a set of divergent thinking tests could increase the predictive efficiency of an established set of cognitive measures. The authors concluded that these additions were worthwhile. However, further investigation was suggested.

Raderman, R., and Allen, D.V. 1974. Registered nurse students in a baccalaureate program: Factors associated with completion. *Nursing Research* 23:71-73.

Selected characteristics of 64 R.N. students who entered a B.S.N. program were compared with characteristics of 33 students who either withdrew or otherwise did not complete the program. Significant differences were found between the two groups in overall GPA, verbal scores on the SAT, NLN Medical-Surgical Examination scores, and type of initial nursing program.

Reece, M.M. 1961. Personality characteristics and success in a nursing program. *Nursing Research* 10:172-176.

The purpose of this study was to determine whether objective measures of personality characteristics are associated with successful completion of a nursing program. Results indicate differences in personality characteristics between the successful nursing students and college women in general, and between students who voluntarily or involuntarily withdrew from training and those who completed the course. Students who withdrew were higher on achievement, autonomy, succorance and dominance but lower on deference, abasement, nurturance and endurance. These students' scores fell between the completed group and the norms for female college students on most items. High ability students who withdrew had less need for deference or nurturance than did the other students.

Reed, C.L., Feldhusen, J.F., and Van Mondfrans, A.P. 1972. Prediction of grade point averages in nursing schools using second-order multiple regression models. *Journal of Educational Measurement* 9(3):181-187.

A study of predictions of first year grade point averages of associate degree nursing students. The primary objective was to determine whether the inclusion of quadratic and/or interaction terms in a regression model would improve the prediction. Results indicate that interaction and quadratic terms improved both the predictability of grade point averages and the replicability of these predictions. The inclusion of higher order terms in prediction research is suggested as a means of improving predictive efficiency.

Reed, C.L., Feldhusen, J.F., and Van Mondfrans, A.P. 1973. Prediction of grade point averages using cognitive and noncognitive predictor variables. *Psychological Reports* 32(1):143-148.

This study investigated the use of noncognitive variables to improve predictions of nursing students' grade point averages. When noncognitive variables were added to an established battery of cognitive predictors, a significant increment to prediction of grade point averages was found.

Rubin, H.S., and O'Mahoney, M.T. 1972. Assessment of attrition-risk populations in nursing education. *Psychological Reports* 31(2):439-442.

Freshman nursing students in a 3-year diploma program were tested by a battery of achievement aptitude, demographic, and personality measures. Product-moment correlations and multiple linear regression were utilized to assess relationships between criterion measures of success, academic failure, and nonacademic withdrawal with personal measures. It is suggested that results may be used to develop an epidemiology of student attrition.

INDEX